CAPTIVE NO MORE

FREEDOM FROM YOUR PAST OF PAIN, SHAME AND GUILT

DR. SCOTT SILVERII

CONTENTS

Copyright v
Introduction xi

1. Freedom From Your Past — 1
2. What is Personal Pain? — 3
3. Why Don't We Deal With the Pain of Our Past? — 7
4. Ways We Manage to Avoid Managing Pain — 13
5. How Our Past Pain Influences Our Present and Future — 19
6. What Is Spiritual Freedom? — 25
7. Live To Forgive and Be Forgiven — 31
8. Inner Vows — 35
9. Judgments — 41
10. Unforgiveness — 47
11. Soul Scars — 53
12. Unseen Enemies — 61
13. Spiritual Oppression — 67
14. Baggage — 73
15. How to Remain Spiritually Free — 77
16. Distorted Image of God — 83
17. Distorted Self-Image — 89
18. Wrong Relationships — 95
19. Unhealthy Personality Traits — 101
20. Anger and Hostility — 107
21. Depression — 115
22. Addiction — 121
23. Armored for Spiritual Warfare — 127
24. Your Daily Walk — 133
25. A Transformed Mind — 139
26. Accountability — 145
27. Boundaries — 151
28. Consequences — 157
29. Restoration — 161
30. Remaining Free — 165

Dr. Scott Silverii 171
Also by Dr. Scott Silverii 173
Paying It Forward 175
Acknowledgments 177

© 2021 *Scott Silverii*

All rights reserved. No part of this publication may be reproduced, distributed, or transmitted in any form or by any means, including photocopying, recording, or other electronic or mechanical methods, without the prior written permission of the publisher, except in the case of brief quotations embodied in critical reviews and certain other noncommercial uses permitted by copyright law. For permission requests, contact Five Stones Press or Dr. Scott Silverii

All Scripture quotations, unless otherwise indicated, are taken from the New American Standard Bible, ©1960, 1962, 1963, 1968, 1971, 1972, 1973, 1975, 1977, 1995 by The Lockman Foundation. Used by permission.

Other versions used are:

KJV—King James Version. Authorized King James Version.

NIV—Scripture taken from the Holy Bible, New International Version®. Copyright © 1973, 1978, 1984 by International Bible Society. Used by permission of Zondervan Publishing House. All rights reserved.

First Edition

Cover Design: Wicked Smart Designs

Editorial Team: Imogen Howsen

Interior Formatting: Five Stones Press Design Team

Publisher: Five Stones Press, Dallas, Texas

For quantity sales, textbooks, and orders by trade bookstores or wholesalers contact Five Stones Press at publish@fivestonespress.net

Five Stones Press is owned and operated by Five Stones Church, a nonprofit 501c3 religious organization. Press name and logo are trademarked. Contact publisher for use.

Dr. Scott Silverii's website is scottsilverii.com

Printed in the United States of America

"A man's got to have a code, a creed to live by, no matter his job."

— JOHN WAYNE

This is to everyone who thought they couldn't go on, but did. This is also to everyone who thinks they can't go on, but will. You are not alone!

INTRODUCTION

The barroom was on the outskirts of a small, mostly forgotten town. I'd shoved a baggie of cocaine in one pocket and had about thirty different pills crammed into another pocket with my stash of weed.

It wasn't enough though. I needed more. I was out of town and all alone. Closing time and the big, outlaw behind the bar began running everyone off. He knew I was looking to score, but would he hook me up me or kick me out like the rest of the junkies?

It was just us. The music had been cranked up with death metal so that my ears felt like there was blood running from them. There was no need for talk. He nodded, and I followed him into this disgusting, one-seater toilet. I'm six-feet-one, but my eyes leveled at the giant's chest. He was massive. I heard the zip of his Buck knife escape the leather sheath strapped to his thigh.

My heart pounded at the reality that we were going to war inside of a rickety plywood potty. All I wanted was to score meth, but I realized the script had been flipped. Still, I didn't care about what might happen. I just needed something to dull the pain.

He dug the sharp tip of the knife's razor's edge into a big bag of that good old, dirty brown stuff. It was crank, and it was what I'd been looking for the whole night.

"Taste it," he demanded.

There was no way I was going to lick that blade. It wasn't a gesture of trust or favor. It was a trap. That crap-hole stall got even smaller as it got more intense. All I wanted was that scoop of meth, but it looked like it was going to cost me my life. Honestly, I didn't care. It was just another of the many times I was forced to fight for my life because of drugs. I was simply exhausted with it all. I carried a piece with me but wedging my hand to grab the snub nose revolver would've been impossible to do without having been carved up like a turkey by his serrated blade. Honestly, I didn't care either way. I just wanted the pain to stop.

I nodded to a small cellophane wrapper, and he snorted like an angry bull before dumping the crank into it.

"I owe you," I whispered through dry lips with the pulse-pumping anticipation of opening up that baggie.

"Yeah, you do," he grunted.

Those were his last words as I stiff-legged it out of that redneck hole-in-the-wall. I still recall how hard it was to walk out of there. My skin tingled and it felt like a cold snake had shivered its slimy way along my spine. Had my thighbones not felt like they'd melted inside my skin, I would've run out there to my truck just to peel the bag open.

I recall swerving my rusted old junker through the dead of night along unlit country back roads. I didn't have a clue where I was or where I was going. All I could focus on was what it meant to have pockets filled with what I needed to put a bandage on the wounds that haunted me daily. Then I saw it. The sign pointing to the bridge that would take me back across the Mississippi River and away from where I knew I had no business medaling.

I smashed my tattered leather boot against the accelerator and the tail end swung wide as dirt spun behind me where it transitioned to asphalt. As my hands shuffled to correct the slide, I laughed at having gotten away with it yet one more time. I promised myself as I glared into the busted up rearview mirror that I'd change. The next day I was going to stop taking these risks just to ease the hurt I felt. It wasn't watering eyes that stopped me from recognizing the man in that reflection. My shaved head and gnarly, oversized beard made me almost unrecognizable. But things would change. I promised. Starting the next day.

My glance into the mirror showed a liquid night sky washed in flashing strobes of blue lights. It was blinding and immediate. There was nowhere to go. Before I could make it to the state line, I was emptying out the contents of my pockets onto the trunk of a police car.

Almost nine months later I returned to the courthouse that subpoenaed me because of those drugs. I'd put on my best suit and tie because it was important to make a good impression for the judge. He was in charge that day, and no matter who I was or what I wanted to do, he would make life-changing decisions.

To be honest, although I'd made a vow to get help and stop living life on the razor's jagged edge, the last nine months were a blur. My personal pain and past haunted me with increasing intensity. I'd continued in a world of guns, drugs and extreme violence. Why? Because it was where I felt most comfortable. The people that roamed that realm where like me and understood that living the white picket fence dream was just that – a dream. Hurting people like me didn't deserve to live in a decent environment. We belonged just where I was—trapped in a nightmare of personal darkness.

So, whether it was this courthouse on that day, or any of the others I'd been demanded to appear in to answer for charges of guns or drugs, it was yet another reminder that I failed to change the vicious cycle of my life.

The prosecuting attorney saw me sitting in the galley with everyone else. I guess I kinda stuck out. I didn't look nice, or kind or patient. And according to most who knew me, they'd say I wasn't. He motioned for me to approach the bench, and my gut started to roil. What now? I kept an eye on the judge as I approached. He didn't seem too impressed, but he was the one who called me there, so it was best to keep quiet as the older man strained to lean over the big wooden divide between he and those to whom he dispensed justice.

Introduction

"You here about the drugs?" the judge asked.

"Yes, sir," I whispered.

My eyes skirted the courtroom. It almost felt like a trap. The same type of trap I'd found myself in the last time I was in the crapper with that outlaw. What was it about this town?

"Well, Special Agent Silverii, looks like you made a trip for nothing. The defendant took a plea deal this morning," said the judge.

A plea deal? I risked my life as an undercover drug agent and all this drug dealing outlaw got was a plea deal. It was code for a slap on the wrist.

"Yes, sir," I said between lips drawn back so tight they felt like splitting in two.

"Thank you for your service," he smiled as he reached across the bench to shake hands.

"My honor, judge."

Tears streamed as I pulled onto the interstate for the five-hour drive back to my office. Punching the inside of the roof to my undercover police vehicle, I was furious with myself. I knew that while I was sentenced to continued suffering, the outlaw was going to get the treatment he probably needed for his own addictions. I was too afraid to ask for help because of what others might think and that I might be seen as weak in my profession.

Over the course of a 25-year law enforcement career, I spent 12 years working undercover and 16 years in SWAT. I was in so much personal pain for most of my adult life, that the only times I felt alive were when my life was most at risk.

These stories might make for exciting TV drama, but they are a horrible way to live your life. Honestly, my suffering didn't start with pinning on a badge. It was much earlier. I learned the truth of past personal pain and how destructive it was. I've also learned how to break free from those chains that shackle us to the darkness of whatever it was that hurt us.

I'd labeled myself as broken and good for nothing but chasing down violent criminals like a predator. I knew it took one to catch one. In my heart, I was falling apart because I'd lost my marriage and

Introduction

family. In my head, I wanted to change, but ego and anger stopped me from doing it. But why?

I was guilty, dead, and buried in my sin, but I was too stubborn to stop and surrender to Christ. While my professional career skyrocketed like a stellar LinkedIn profile, my personal life remained mired in rejection, abandonment, addiction, and consistently crappy choices.

The kicker about sin is while we can be restored if we repent and ask forgiveness, there are still consequences. Some consequences take the form of alimony, child support, or a rental home while joint property is liquidated. Others attack our ego—public exposure, humiliation, loss of respect and career. Still others have a more serious and permanent effect such as addictions, disease, and death.

My troubles didn't start with my job. They began as a kid. I grew up Godless, in the shadow of a dominant, detached father. His physical intimidation and control through silence left me without ever having heard a kind word, seeing an interest in my life, or speaking the words, "I love you."

Family dysfunction screws up a lot of us, and the messed-up part is that we go years without a clue that how we were raised wasn't the way things were supposed to be. All we know is what we know. But that doesn't make it right. It just makes us hurt. To this day there is nothing I could've done to prevent or change history. But I did have the opportunity to define my response in the present. I decided to heal, and then God led me to share so you can heal too.

In case you were wondering what happened after that undercover case was done, and the hundreds of others that followed, I never sought out help. I sprinted from one high-risk investigation to the next. Eventually I placed myself into a coffin called guilt, held a funeral called pain, and buried myself in a grave called shame. It wasn't until God's mercy and grace raised me up, brushed me off, and gave me the key to freedom from my past that I was able to live again.

I live the life of "Leave No One Behind." I'm here for you. *Freedom From Your Painful Past* is my way of paying it forward. God has been so merciful when all I wanted to do was end it. His grace and blessings

Introduction

have shown that there is light in life and that we were not created to suffer, but to celebrate being His! Walk with me and I promise to show you the truths about what has latched itself onto your back, and most importantly, how to free yourself from it.

Rak Chazak Amats!!!
Scott

1

FREEDOM FROM YOUR PAST

So if the Son sets you free, you will be free indeed.
John 8:36

I'm so thankful you've joined me here at *Captive No More*. If you have been or are still trapped in the bondage of pain, shame and guilt from something in your past, this is where we work together to gain permanent freedom.

For decades, I struggled with the effects of past pain. I knew nothing about the reality that pain carried forward, or that it would continue to create problems in my life. I mistakenly figured what was in the past was in the past. If problems lingered, then it was my problem for not getting over it, or even worse, being soft.

Although in my head I wanted to change, I didn't have the tools to make it happen. I knew I was hurting and eventually began to accept the fact that I must be broken and of no value. I had allowed my past to define my present and the curse of pain to steal the joy of freedom.

When we talk about pain, we first think of physical pain from injury or accident. There is a self-reliant, internal block on the notion of our emotions or feelings being hurt. How could they be, we're after all! Now, don't worry because I'm not going to get tree hugger on you, but it would be a waste of your time if we didn't dig into everything.

That was my stubborn mindset for years but thank God for the revelation that my unresolved pain was devastating and held a lasting effect on my life. Even more thanks that God showed me how to free myself from the stranglehold of what living a life of hurt and hate had caused.

I was blessed by His mercy and want to share God's Word and my journey toward liberation from what had destroyed so much of me for so many years. We're here together to make major changes in our lives, so I wanted to make sure *Freedom From Your Past Pain* has a maximum impact. Let's commit to making this happen. Our other friends have found that it works best if you commit to carving out time daily to pray over this, read each day's message, and respond to the Call To Action sections.

Here's to you finding freedom from your past.

Scott

Call To Action

1. Write out what you think is meant by past personal pain.

2. Write out a list of what past pains still hurt you.

3. Write out a list of anyone who has caused you to hurt in your past.

4. Write out a detailed example of how a past pain still causes struggle today.

2

WHAT IS PERSONAL PAIN?

Now the Lord is the Spirit, and where the Spirit of the Lord is, there is freedom.
2 Corinthians 3:17

Identifying past pain, for us men, is usually a tough job. It's like that itch you just can't seem to scratch or the word on the tip of your tongue. It's there and has an effect on you, but it's nothing you can touch, taste or tangibly describe. Whatever it is, it's just there.

Now on the other hand, if the pain you carry is from a source you clearly recall, then the memory may be very present, but the extent of how it affects you may not be so evident. Despite the variations of our personal experiences with past pain, we have a horrible habit of not addressing it.

Before we begin to dig down to discover the source of our own hurt, I'm going to do you a huge favor by telling you about a lie that almost all of us have been fed. It's also something we've clung to it as if it's the gospel truth. You ready?

Time does NOT heal all wounds.

There, I said it. While it may not have instantly changed your life, it is an important block on which we'll build this challenge for gaining freedom. Why is it so important? Because it's what we as a culture have accepted, and there's an unrealistic expectation for time to actually heal all wounds.

I've spent decades wondering what was ailing me. I thought I was weak because I carried guilt from things I had done in my past. I lugged around shame for feeling sadness, hurt, and anger about stuff that also happened in my past. I say junk because that's what it is today. It's just junk that I had no control over back then, and it has no value in my life now. It's junk, and like any pile of trash if it isn't properly disposed of, it'll rot until becoming unbearable.

We're not going to wait on time to heal anything. This is where we take action and work hard to gain our own healing through the restorative power and grace of Jesus Christ.

So, what is past pain, and how exactly are we going to work toward being freed from it? That's a great start and defining what it is will be your personal journey. Getting and staying away from it is where we work together to get there.

Sources and causes for our past pain may result from cases of neglect, abuse, abandonment, parents' divorce, our own divorce, broken relationships, traumatic loss or death, being bullied, school issues, self-esteem, puberty, sexual identity, gender confusion, serious illness or disease, or any of the many things that get under our skin and clamp down until we feel as though we've lost control.

It's important that if you haven't already identified what it is that haunts you, to really begin praying over this. Ask God to reveal to you want it is in your spirit that you need to be freed from. These bonds that tether us to past events, and people are called soul ties.

As soon as he had finished speaking to Saul, the soul of Jonathan was knit to the soul of David, and Jonathan loved him as his own soul.
1 Samuel 18:1

While soul ties can be positive bonds to old friends and family, they are also spiritual attachments to events, actions, images or anything that trapped you in that moment in time that just won't allow you to be free to move forward with your life.

Some people visualize these spiritual ties as strands, like spiderwebs that stretch from that moment in the past to where they are today. When I began to understand the concept of soul ties, I immediately saw my past pain connected to my spirit by giant suspension bridge cables.

It might sound funny if this is your first exposure to the reality of soul ties, but once you begin to pray over them, you will start to "see" yourself still physically connected to your past. Like I said, mine were so powerfully destructive over the course of my life that they were like thick, impenetrable cables. But, as I prayed God's authority over them, they were sliced like a hot knife through butter.

Too often, we just blow it off. Most of us don't like going to a doctor when we're sick or hurt because we figure it'll go away or we can just deal with it. Past, personal pain is the same way. Can you live with guilt and shame? Sure, you can…until you can't.

Outside of suicide, which is our final, most desperate effort to stop the hurting, we turn to medicating the negative effects. Consider your own methods of dealing with harmful issues. While not everything we do is as destructive as suicide, the effort is often driven by a need to ease the injury.

I'll give you an example of someone you know. Me.

I grew up in a home dominated by my very intimidating father. He never said he loved me, or liked me, or for that matter, never anything even nice. I grew up telling myself that he was just the strong, silent type of father who showed his love instead of expressing it. I also didn't realize how his rejection affected my entire life.

The pain I carried with me for decades dominated my life and the decisions I made without me ever understanding what was going on. I know of people in their eighties who are recovering from childhood hurts that sting as deep as if it had just occurred.

The point is, we can muddle through life never scratching that itch, or we can rid ourselves of it, and move forward with living the blessed life that God created for us.

Call To Action

1. Write out everything you understand to be a negative soul tie in your life.

2. Write out in detail everything that you are aware of that has caused you past pain.

3. Write out a pledge to cut yourself free from the tethers of negative soul ties and forgive those who have hurt you in the past.

3
WHY DON'T WE DEAL WITH THE PAIN OF OUR PAST?

"I have the right to do anything," you say—but not everything is beneficial. "I have the right to do anything"—but I will not be mastered by anything.
1 Corinthians 6:12

Many years ago, before I retired from law enforcement, I commanded a large, nationally accredited investigations bureau. One case in particular required all of the resources of my division. Detectives, juvenile investigators, narcotics agents and SWAT were all rallied together to solve this case. Although we knew without a doubt the person was guilty of heinous crimes, we never made an arrest.

Why?

Because hurt people would rather suffer in silence than face the potential of pain, shame or humiliation by confronting past injuries head-on. This case that still haunts me involved decades of sexual abuse by a man against many young boys. As we searched for victims to testify, they had all grown to be late teenagers and young men. Although we held documents confirming the sex crimes, not a single one would admit that they'd been sexually molested.

The point is, while not all past pain is caused by sexual abuse, we prefer to hide our dirty laundry. The risk of airing it out to even our most trusted friends or a professional counselor is not worth the risk of losing face in the self-esteem department.

Studies in the United States show men are more likely than women to commit suicide, a ratio of 3.6 to 1. This isn't just an American tragedy. Worldwide, men terminate themselves much more often than women.

Let's take a look at some of the deeper reasons we avoid exposing pain to a healing light. Of course, our culture encourages "real men" to endure as much pain as humanly possible without showing it. To do so would be to show weakness and be considered much less of a man. Woman, who hurt just as deeply, seem to be more open to seeking and receiving help.

Like I said, that is the culture in which we live. The perception is not correct, but it is what we've allowed it to become. So why would we rather crash and burn than heal? To start, most of us are pushed to be fixers and doers. We go to great lengths just to avoid asking for help. It's the way we are genetically inclined.

Before we begin to blame God for creating us this way, the reality of being a fixer and a doer is not a bad thing. It's actually how and why we've survived as a species for centuries. Unfortunately, like too much of a good thing, we allowed humanity to become defined primarily by our ability to fix, do and endure.

We are also driven by ego, a major factor in our help avoidance. The right ego is important to the alpha mindset. An attack on our ego by showing a need for help is interpreted as a diminished capacity. Humility is on very limited display when ego is running the show.

In the years I suffered most, there were people who cared about my well-being. They recognized that I needed help. But, in the public position I held, and operating within an occupational culture of cops, seeking help meant a threat to my esteem, status and definitely my pride.

No thank you to getting help. I defiantly chose to suck it up and reinforce the façade that shielded my weaknesses. While it did allow me to move throughout my career, it came to a tipping point where I knew an implosion was imminent.

Many people don't understand the mentality of *"all and nothing."* People who pursue ways to help them not hate themselves so much must go for it all; there's no happy medium. If/when that ends in a mess, there's no consideration for retooling for repair and recovery. It becomes an issue of nothing.

The reality is, when it implodes into nothing, wounded people are not threatened, afraid or hesitant to commit suicide. The scandal that occurred as their lives collapsed wasn't the problem. The fact that a problem existed that they couldn't handle on their own was the problem. As opposed to enduring the failure of exposure that they couldn't fix it, we rationalize suicide as not only ending their pain, problem and public exposure, but that their broken life wasn't worth the effort of collecting the pieces.

Dominance becomes a major factor in why people, most particularly men, refuse to seek help. There is the misconception that we were placed on this earth to dominate it with an aggressive, conquering iron fist. Genesis gives God's authorization to have dominion over all things on earth. It was also reaffirmed through Noah, but there is no charge to lord over all; but to care for, nurture and multiply. That command to care for also applies to ourselves.

Then God said, "Let us make mankind in our image, in our likeness, so that they may rule over the fish in the sea and the birds in the sky, over the livestock and all the wild animals,
and over all the creatures that move along the ground."
Genesis 1:26

While the previous factors keeping people from seeking help are characteristics we take seriously and are also helpful qualities in life when not taken to extreme, there are other reasons stopping us.

Victimhood implies someone overcame you, and that you were

incapable of defending yourself or others. We see the role of needing protection as that of women, children and the elderly. If we've been victimized, then that shows we weren't strong enough, smart enough or good enough to fight off an attack from a more dominant force. That failure is best hidden in our wounded spirit where the consequences will continue to torment us long after the threat of being the victim has passed.

Failure is not an option for most men. After all, who wants to fail? We place value in our ability to succeed regardless of who it affects or how we define that success. I still recall the television character of Al Bundy. I bet you can tell me how many touchdowns he scored in one football game. Poor guy's greatest success occurred one Friday night decades ago, but that was and remained his definition of success.

Are we stuck in the past because the future holds pain that occurred back then? Are we living our lives below the radar because we know just how fragile we actually are without getting help? Are we so afraid of being seen as a failure that we've chosen to live a lie? Failure is not getting knocked down. It's refusing to get back up.

As I wrap up this section about why we refuse to deal with the pain from our past, I want to circle back to the beginning story of the criminal investigation of the serial child molester.

Not all past pain stems from sexual sin, many do. Whether it's molestation, abuse, rape, pornography, early exposure or experimentation, or a general confusion created by an absence of adult guidance, many experience problems based on these and other issues with sex.

One of the final factors that stop us from seeking help with pain is being seen as less than sexually capable or homosexual. The many victims we'd interviewed during that criminal case were heterosexual and were now married. They had no intention of opening a can of worms that included being illegally sexually assaulted by a man.

Understand that your maturity and mentality level at that age does not define who you are today. Whether it was forced upon you, or you were youthfully curious in your experimentation, the young you does not define the current you. Is there forgiveness and forgiving required? There may be, and if so, you must pursue that. But you are not condemned to live a secreted life of pain, shame and guilt.

God assures us that we are new creations in Christ, and that the old man falls away. There is no need to continue living with darkness hidden in your life. But it will take the healing light of Jesus Christ to begin the healing and restoration of your joy.

Therefore, if anyone is in Christ, he is a new creation; old things have passed away; behold, all things have become new.
2 Corinthians 5:17

Call To Action

1. Write out whether or not you are open to receiving help in healing from past pain. If not, write as if explaining to your most loved ones, why you refuse help to heal.

2. Write out what you would want help in healing to look like.

3. Write out what you see your life as like living without what haunts you.

4

WAYS WE MANAGE TO AVOID MANAGING PAIN

You, my brothers and sisters, were called to be free. But do not use your freedom to indulge the flesh; rather, serve one another humbly in love. For the entire law is fulfilled in keeping this one command: "Love your neighbor as yourself."
Galatians 5:13-14

What's really eating away at you? Are regrets consuming your thoughts so you're forced to constantly shut them down? Can you sit in silence without a mental movie flooding your brain and demanding that you fill the quiet space where unhealthy thoughts roam free?

You're not alone. The pain we carry from our past is tucked away and always available to muck up our lives or turn gold star moments into brown star regrets. We allow pain, shame and regret to overwhelm us with stress over how to cope with it. Unfortunately, the coping solves nothing. Healing does.

Have you developed your own secret way of helping to ease that hurt? Does your way involve something that, if exposed, would embarrass you, ruin your reputation or cost you a career? If so, then you are not working toward healing, you are enabling the hurt.

It's not an uncommon practice for us men. We avoid dealing with all types of pain, from physical ailments to emotional trauma. Is it good for us? Not always, but it's what we do. This is also a practice of avoiding God by not trusting Him to provide for restoration.

Why do we avoid God? Because the devil whispers in our ear that we're not worthy, and that we can't trust God because all He wants to do is convict and punish us. I will tell you that there is no other way to be freed from the pain of your past than through Jesus Christ the great healer and physician.

We also like to weigh risk versus reward before taking action. Hurting people often consider the worst-case scenario, along with how long they can get away with avoiding help from others. God gives us biblical examples and consequences of how avoiding Him only drags out the injury. There are three primary ways we try to manage pain.

DAVID

King David was exalted as a great and mighty ruler. God himself chose David to be king over Israel because of what He saw on the inside. Although David was anointed by God, he didn't come to the throne without serious personal baggage. David is a lot like us in carrying personal pain from our past.

David did as good a job as he could with avoiding what troubled him, but like us, it eventually became too much to bear and soon cost him personally.

> *Man looks at how someone appears on the outside.*
> *But I look at what is in the heart.*
> *1 Samuel 16:7b*

The example of David is used because he engaged in one of the most common ways for dealing with past pain. Instead of addressing what issues in his past caused him so much hurt, David began to medicate his pain.

There are many ways to ease our pain. Some of us use alcohol, drugs, sex, exercise, work, or any of many addictions to compensate for the hurt we feel by an emptiness caused by an unresolved pain.

Because David preferred to seek a temporary fix instead of a permanent solution for his personal injuries, he used what we refer to as **medication** in unsuccessfully dealing with pain. David's medication of choice was the flesh. His sexual addiction caused problems for everyone associated with him. David's family suffered greatly because of his sexual sin, and a generational curse was cast upon his children.

David's pain was rooted in the rejection by his father, Jesse. He wasn't considered worthy of meeting the prophet Samuel, who was sent by God to anoint a ruler. Yet, there in that rejected, messed-up boy, Israel had a king. David's rejection by his father stung and stuck. Have you been hurt by a parent and never forgave them? This injury doesn't heal in time.

I'll share that as a kid, I'd gotten a red warm-up suit with white stripes. It looked just like my hero, Steve Austin, The Six Million Dollar Man. I wore it everywhere.

One day my dad called out to me, but I was mixing it up with the neighborhood kids and didn't hear him. Then his words became very clear, "Hey, idiot in that red suit, I'm talking to you." I was about ten years old. I stuffed that track suit in the trash, and forty-two years later, those words still hurt.

SOLOMON

The son of David, Solomon, was by far the wealthiest and most wise human ever to grace the earth. Despite growing up in a home rocked by the earlier scandal between his father, David, and the sexual affair he had with a married woman, Bathsheba (also his mother), Solomon was loved by God and blessed tremendously.

The generational curse David incurred upon his family because of his failure to address past pain caused personal suffering for his son also. Solomon's wounds as a result of family sin and the shame caused by the sexual affair of his father and mother drove him to compensate in a very different way than David's medication.

Motivation and achievements were Solomon's failed attempt to soothe his pain. The more he accumulated the less he felt deserving. In Ecclesiastes 2 he shares the futility of trying to outwork his hurt.

I've included this small section of the scripture, but please read the entire Chapter 2:1-24.

> *10 I denied myself nothing my eyes desired;*
> *I refused my heart no pleasure.*
> *My heart took delight in all my labor,*
> *and this was the reward for all my toil.*
> *11 Yet when I surveyed all that my hands had done*
> *and what I had toiled to achieve,*
> *everything was meaningless, a chasing after the wind;*
> *nothing was gained under the sun.*
> Ecclesiastes 2:10-11

This is so personal to me, as I suspect it is to many of you. I crushed and conquered my way through a career, athletics and academics to help me feel less empty. It soon became impossible to fill these empty spaces. Avoiding true healing and spiritual freedom through God's grace and mercy dooms us to an unending effort of emptiness and unsatisfactory results.

Our spirit requires peace, not prizes.

ABSOLOM

There is a third unhealthy way of dealing with our hurt. Absalom was David's son and Solomon's half-brother. His pain, like many with a dominant parent, began at home. Absalom also suffered from intense guilt over doing nothing to defend his sister from a sexual attack by another half-brother.

How often do we find ourselves in a situation we know is wrong, yet we sit by as injustice is acted out? Acts of abuse or unfair treatment occurs often among families and friends. Being a victim or witness causes pain that, if not resolved, will continue to fester.

Meditation stewed in Absalom's spirit as hatred intensified. For two years he avoided confronting his feelings and the offender before it erupted, and he killed his half-brother.

Absalom's deep-seated pain directed against his father; David caused him to try overthrowing his reign. Absalom's desire to destroy his own father led to his death. Attacks against others is what defines Absalom. Are you feeling the rage of regret and wrongdoings roil beneath the surface while you look for an outlet to unleash your fury upon?

Which One Are You?

Do you booze it until you lose it, yet things are worse than they began? Please understand that the substances used to fight addiction are not the problem. The problem is you're using addictive substances to avoid healing from your pain.

Brothers and sisters; drinking, screwing and fighting will not heal your hurt. Don't listen to the devil. You are good and you are worthy to be loved. God wants to heal you because He loves you. He's not waiting to smack you like a carnival game of whack-a-mole.

Allow yourself to heal. It's better than the hurt.

God placed a message on my heart that remains with me today. "Avoiding is not winning." You can only sweep so much junk under the rug. If it's confessing a wrong to a friend, spouse, co-worker, or forgiving yourself for messing up once again, time does not heal all wounds. It is a lie, so don't let pain fester in your life.

Call To Action

1.Write out which of the three examples are you most like (Medication, Motivation or Meditation)

2.Write out ways you've developed to ease or cope with your past pain.

3.Write out the personal, professional and social consequences if someone exposed your coping mechanisms.

5
HOW OUR PAST PAIN INFLUENCES OUR PRESENT AND FUTURE

But Scripture has locked up everything under the control of sin, so that what was promised, being given through faith in Jesus Christ, might be given to those who believe.
Galatians 3:22

I don't think there is any disagreement about whether our earlier life plays a role for influencing who we are today. Not only do genetics through DNA influence us on an individual level, but society, culture and experiences play important roles in shaping who we are.

We're out of luck changing our DNA, but we have God's full authority to become redefined in His light through Jesus Christ. Now, with that encouraging piece of information, let's look at what and why we might want to make changes to who we are, and how we came to be that way.

> *Therefore, if anyone is in Christ,*
> *the new creation has come:*
> *The old has gone, the new is here!*
> *2 Corinthians 5:17*

Going back to our earliest days of childhood, bad experiences can and usually do have a lingering or profound effect on how you behave as an adult. Dysfunctional family dynamics are the most common cause of persistent adult pain. Unhappiness or trauma during a child's most formative years has the potential for causing tremendous scarring for the adult.

Maybe it was an alcoholic parent, or a family member who subjected others to physical, mental or sexual abuse. Parents suffering with depression leave impressions of abandonment on their kids although they may be physically in the same home.

Past pain can and often does push beyond emotional barriers until it affects you physically, psychologically and spiritually. This surrounding of turmoil also creates an unhealthy environment for those related or associated with you.

Unrecognized past personal pain may evolve into chronic mental disorders such as states of depression, anxiety and PTSD (post-traumatic stress disorder.) Living in a state of chaos, whether real or perceived, places the brain in a red zone of self-defense. Do you feel like no one likes or respects you? How about the feelings that your job is in jeopardy or that someone is trying to take your position away from you?

I'm not talking about wearing a tinfoil hat while taping newspapers over your windows, but I am talking about the effects of darkness in your life. Without realizing it, you may be placing your job, your marriage or your family at risk. If your pain is driving you to drinking, drug use, porn consumption, or any number of reactions beyond what is healthy, then you might just have someone after you and your job.

The reality is that while you are compressed beneath the pressure of darkness in your spirit caused by pain, your instincts may have become dulled by the persistent internal agony. Your brain will also rewire as a result of the constant state of discomfort. Through the process of neuroplasticity, the brain protects and prepares itself based on past and current data.

Once you are aware that there is an issue, although you may not know what it is or where it began, you can be sure that your body has already begun the transformative process of self-preservation. This is why it's so important at this point where you've made a commitment to heal, that you must follow through on that effort.

There are an unlimited number of scenarios with the potential for causing harm to you as a child. There are also varying degrees of severity for how any one or a combination of several factors influence who you are as an adult. The important thing to remember is that you are not to blame for what happened as a child, but you are responsible for how you choose to react to it as an adult.

We're here working together to understand why you continue to act out in a way that is harmful for you and possibly embarrassing as well. The majority of time, your irregular behavior, thoughts and emotions can be traced back to trauma experienced in childhood. But let's also consider that pain experienced as an adult is just as influential as harm known as a child.

Sometimes the injuries are even more severe and impactful because we add the caveat of guilt for not knowing better as an adult or having been victimized by a trusted person. There is the added shame of being duped or hurt by another peer seen as your equal. So, you see, no one is immune to being harmed, but we can improve our ability to be restored if we focus on the healing instead of the hurt.

Let's consider the person who was cheated on or abandoned by their spouse or someone they loved dearly. The thoughtless acts of an unfaithful partner do leave scars. It may also cause you to no longer trust the opposite sex because you see them as cruel, so you either avoid commitment or hurt them before they hurt you. Whether or not they ever intended to hurt you, that is.

While childhood harm causes fear and instability, adult damage attacks confidence and self-esteem. Compensation often takes a form of behavior that becomes as self-destructive as the core cause. You can think through the ways we compensate and how that influences who you are and how you behave.

Is it uncommon for the child of an alcoholic to become an alcoholic, or a wife beater to abuse his own spouse? How about men who were sexually abused and grow up with intimacy issues, gender confusion or struggles with homo or bisexuality.

Once you drop the guarded defense of your behavior and stop making excuses, you will begin to identify particular behaviors that are traceable to a point in the past. Whether that point was decades or weeks ago, it doesn't matter. What does matter is that you have the God-given authority to change that behavior by working to heal what has hurt you.

I'll end this with something wonderful that happened through my own healing. My wife had grown weary of a habit I had, but never realized I was doing it. Anytime she reached out to touch me, I would either block it (gently) with a self-defense type technique or quickly pull away. She took that as me rejecting her pursuit and affection.

Her love language is touch, and like many women, she needs non-intimate touching throughout the day to reinforce the feeling of security which leads to intimacy. Instead, I'd turned us into a set of sparring partners with the only touching being my horseplay, or during sex.

Once God began to reveal the core cause of my defensive behavior, I understood that I was overly protective of being touched because intimacy, gentleness and loving attention was not given to me as a child. I saw physical contact as a threat to harm, direct or control. Those associations kept my body in a state of constant tension and alarm.

Eventually, as God began healing the hurt I'd carried around for decades, I was able to let down my guard and allow my wife in. Emotional, physical and spiritual abandonment is common in the childhood lives of many grown men. The conflict is made more confusing when the parent(s) are in the home, but still avoid the familial connect.

If you are continuing to struggle with current behavior or acting out but don't know why, this is the perfect time to seek your God goggles to re-examine your life to see the truth from your past. God isn't going to judge you for it.

Dig deep into who you were to find out who you are. Please remember you don't have to continue to be that person The apostle Paul made it a daily practice to forget those things which are behind, so that he could reach forward to pursue the life God blessed him with. Time to move forward.

"...but one thing I do, <u>forgetting those things which are behind</u> and reaching forward to those things which are ahead. I press toward the goal for the prize of the upward call of God in Christ Jesus."
Philippians 3:12

Call To Action
1. Write out in detail one painful memory from your childhood.
2. Write out in detail one painful event from adulthood.
3. Write out how each of these may continue to be present and influence your behavior.
4. Write out a statement of commitment that releases you from the events and frees you to heal from all remnants of them.

6

WHAT IS SPIRITUAL FREEDOM?

It is for freedom that Christ has set us free. Stand firm, then, and do not let yourselves be burdened again by a yoke of slavery.
Galatians 5:1

There are many definitions and descriptions for helping us to explain spiritual freedom. In the context of freedom from your past personal pain, let's talk about what it looks like for us, men.

Past pain is harbored in the darkness of our hearts. We may not even realize it's hidden there, but this is why we're working together to identify it, and root it out. Let's assume you have either recognized you have an issue with baggage from your past that is interfering with your present, or you have that persistent bug in your ear that something's just not right in your life.

Either of these are safe assumptions because you've invested in this challenge and are committed to slicing through the chains holding you down. While you can enjoy an intimate relationship with God through the salvation of Jesus Christ, there is still work to be done on clearing out the dark chambers in your heart. This is where resistance, pride and pain reside.

The only way to eliminate darkness is by exposing it to light. The light of Christ is the remedy for the dark pain that still causes you to stumble, sin and separate yourself from God's loving will. Too many of us think that our pain is too deep to heal, but if you believe in God, then you know there is nothing, and I mean absolutely nothing, that He cannot do.

You can know spiritual freedom from the negative effects of past personal pain. God didn't create you to live a life below the radar. He loves you and wants you to know Him on an intimate level, so that you'll trust Him enough to pursue His will for your life. The spiritual freedom is a condition where past problems with continuing shame, blame and guilt prevent you from being comfortable in God's presence.

Being free also means you are confident to openly live for God and exist in a state of transparency, trust and accountability. This isn't to say that your business becomes everyone else's business, but a forgiving nature that is also forgiven allows you to move freely without the fear of exposure.

A fantastic guy I knew for years confided in me one day that his life was junk. I was and wasn't shocked. He was a leader and mentor. He'd been so good to me throughout my career, that although I looked up to him as a boss, I knew something was off.

Aaron, I'll call him, spoke with me one day after I'd moved on to another agency. He said it would have been odd having the conversation while he was officially my supervisor. I understood, but it hurt me to know that he'd not only struggled but also felt he had to conceal his pain for the sake of status.

Aaron was past the end of his rope when he finally decided to seek help. He'd struggled because of neglect and abandonment. His life was full of emptiness and a constant feeling of not being good enough. That feeling was the driving force behind his obsession to achieve rank throughout his career. But, no matter how much money and professional status he earned, he said it was never enough.

Although in public he was respected and enjoyed many friends, he lived in darkness and was so ashamed of what he did behind closed doors. Aaron said that if ever exposed, he planned to kill himself to save the embarrassment.

I completely understood where he was coming from. It's not uncommon to live with an emptiness that is never filled. We try to cram that hole with promotions, money, thrill seeking, sex, parting or living a life on a bigger scale than anyone else. But at the end of each and every day, we go to bed even more alone and disappointed than when the day began.

Aaron said he knew he was messed up, but no matter how hard he tried to do better, he kept making the same mistakes and getting lower and lower in life. He was quite honest about his plan to commit suicide. He admitted that he felt he still had a life to live for, but he was sick of the rut he couldn't escape from. He knew he was a better person but didn't understand why he couldn't act like a better person in his private life.

Aaron saw his inability to move in a positive direction as a personal failure because he couldn't "fix" himself. In many men's lives, failure isn't an option they're willing to carry for long. It goes back to us being doers and fixers. Aaron could do it and he could fix it, and just like us, all he needed was a little help.

Like me, Aaron knew there was a problem, but he just couldn't put his finger on it. Once I understood that my current problems stemmed from past pain, I was able to finally realize that:

1. I didn't create the original problem
2. I wasn't responsible for what was done to me then, but I am responsible for what I do for me now.
3. I am not defined nor condemned by my past.
4. God gives me the authority to free myself from past personal pain.
5. God grants me the grace and blessing to live a blessed life.

Once I found peace in these truths, I began to peer deep into my past with what I called God Goggles. My mind, heart and head were open to the reality of re-examining my past. Not only things done to me, but also things I'd done. We gain a Christlike understanding when we pray for spiritual freedom from the chains that hold us in darkness.

Part of that new understanding is seeing things in truth. Coming to accept the truth in events, we are also able to accept that there is an accountability and potential consequences not only for the harm from others, but harm caused by us.

As I led Aaron through these early stages of revelation, he began to shudder at what was shown to him about his past. Events he participated in but were always minimized as youthful indiscretions, were now understood as violent and sometimes criminal acts. He began to experience a breaking open within his soul. He'd never felt empathy for others or himself.

God was drip-feeding Aaron glimpses from his past. They were like rain drops on parched earth. The more Aaron prayed to be revealed to him, the more his spirit opened up to receive the truth about not only the things he did while acting out of anger and hurt, but the harmful things done to him that he'd suppressed or denied.

Soon, Aaron's life as he'd defined it had been toiled up like the lifeless, cracked soil of his past. But, although it hurt, he remained faithful and hungry to know more about what held such a stranglehold on his life. Eventually, spiritual freedom planted the seeds of truth in his soul, and they began to bud and blossom into a once dark past now exposed and completely open for God to shine in His healing light.

Aaron chose life over death and continued to pursue Christ as his source of light and life. He's remarried, loves being a dad, and continues to thrive in his career. The big difference is that Aaron lives life in the openness of God's spiritual freedom from past pain.

Call To Action

1. Write out a prayer for healing from past pain.

2. Write out what issues still remain in the dark chambers of your heart.

3. Have you surrendered everything to Christ? If not, write out what you are trying to hide and why is it so important to you.

7

LIVE TO FORGIVE AND BE FORGIVEN

In him and through faith in him we may approach God with freedom and confidence.
Ephesians 3:12

As we move forward in the process to heal from our past pain, it's important that we consider how valuable the ability to forgive is in the process. Many men, myself included, spent many years not understanding what true forgiveness meant. We saw forgiveness as weakness. We looked at a sin or harm committed against us, and wondered how could we possibly let the violator off of the hook for what they did to us?

Forgiveness is not about agreeing to or approving of what the violator did to us. Forgiving others is about setting ourselves free. Forgiveness allows us to be free from not only the person, but the acts that hurt us.

It's easy to continue harboring hard feelings against someone who hurt us, but that anger is like poison we ingest while trying to hurt someone else. God is very clear about His demand that we forgive others. He carries it a step further and declares that if we fail to forgive others, He will not forgive us. Talk about motivation to come into a position of humble surrender! No grudge I held was ever worth so much as to separate myself from God.

> *For if you forgive others their trespasses, your heavenly Father will also forgive you. But if you do not forgive others, then your Father will not forgive your trespasses.*
> *Matthew 6:14-16*

So, what's this business about forgiving? It took me years of harboring grudges, hard feelings, and hatred toward others before I came to understand the blessing of forgiveness. Like many others, I might've said, "I forgive you" to someone just to get past whatever it was that made me angry or hurt, but that was just paying lip service to them.

The truth of forgiving is that it's not for pacifying others. It is about our obedience to God's desire to live Christ-like. It's also about mirroring God's response to sin by forgiving us, so that we may separate the interference that unconfessed and unforgiven sin creates.

A guy I mentored that we'll call Chuck, had a longstanding feud with his siblings. As their mother drew closer to death, the brothers' and sisters' infighting grew more intense, and the potential for physical harm escalated. As so many families experience, once she passed, they all began to fight over unspecified elements of their mother's will. It got bad; really bad.

After about two years, and no settlement, Chuck reached out to me for help. His health was diminishing, his marriage was falling apart, and his faith was tested beyond anything he'd known.

I saw it in his face. He had to forgive his family. His initial reaction was what you can imagine. "No way. Do you know what they did to me?"

Yes, I knew exactly what they did to him. They hurt and disrespected him. For a man, respect is the language we speak. Most of us don't mind talking, discussing or arguing, but once the other person becomes disrespectful; it's over. Chuck was over it; except he was still suffering from the fallout.

He may not have been engaged in the arguments or relationships anymore, but he was still very much involved. He was tied to them through an unforgiving spirit. Instead of freedom, he was trapped by them and he was also separated from God's will and blessings. He looked completely isolated.

Chuck needed to know the truth, and he needed to put it into action immediately. His life depended on it. I shared the biblical truths of forgiveness and God's command to mirror His and His Son's forgiving nature. Chuck was so wounded that he actually said he could never, ever forgive his siblings. He said it would take a miracle. What it would take was faith.

I assured him that God already knew his heart and He wanted to hear Chuck's voice. He didn't even have to tell his siblings that he forgave them in person, he just needed to speak the words. Chuck said he began in his shower, and in his car while he was alone. He'd say their names and that he forgave them. But to be honest, he said he didn't believe it.

After about a week, Chuck said each time he'd say a sibling's name in prayer, his anger at the sound of the name became less. He began to feel compassion for each one as God placed the realities of why they acted out the way they did. In that, he also saw reasons from his past where pain drove his behavior toward them.

Eventually, Chuck said God placed the grace of mercy and forgiveness for his siblings in his heart, and immediately, Chuck noticed the hatred he carried had disappeared. He didn't know when it left, but he knew his heart was free. Soon, he was able to pray blessings over each sibling.

Chuck was at a point of seamless submission to God's will, and then he had a decision to make. He'd experienced the transition through forgiving and blessing without ever having to speak with his offending siblings. Now, he began to consider the possibility of restoring a relationship with them. God allows us authority when we forgive. We're not trapped with the offender, nor are we forced to endure their actions and behavior.

We can fully forgive someone, yet still have the authority to never speak with them again. I use the term pruning. In life there are relationships that suck positive, life giving energy away from you and ruin the possibility of new, nurturing relationships.

Although he fully forgave them, Chuck chose to end the relationships with his siblings because their lives were filled with chaos and unteachable spirits that threatened the peace in faith God granted him. Chuck said God removed the desire for those relationships, and though he prays each comes to know Christ, he understands that he's not the one to lead them to Him.

You might be asking what happened with all of the money and possessions that were stolen by Chuck's siblings. I helped him to understand that it was not his duty to punish his siblings for their sins. They sinned against God by violating His laws. We have no authority to police on behalf of God. He's fully capable of handling violators on His own. Matter of fact, I'd much prefer God handle it.

Avenge not yourselves, beloved, but give place unto the wrath of God: for it is written, Vengeance belongeth unto me;
I will recompense, saith the Lord.
Romans 12:19

So how does this relate to us, men? We will not, and I repeat, we will not ever know freedom from our past until we forgive those who have sinned against us. Forgiving is Freeing.

Call To Action

1. Write out 3 people whom you hold a grudge, hate or anger toward.
2. Write out in detail what each of those people did that hurt you.
3. Write out their name, and the words, "I forgive you."

8

INNER VOWS

"Therefore, my friends, I want you to know that through Jesus the forgiveness of sins is proclaimed to you. Through him everyone who believes is set free from every sin, a justification you were not able to obtain under the law of Moses.
Acts 13:38-39

Inner vows are common among most men. We make them as boys, teens and young men. They range from what we'll be when we grow up to who we'll marry to what type of job we'll secure.

While these can be harmless aspirations and life goals, the critical point is when they become destructive because of the emotional framework being erected outside of God's will for our life.

Let's take a quick step back and define just what an inner vow is so we're on the same page. According to Pastor Jimmy Evans, from his book *Freedom From Your Past*, they are a self-oriented commitment made in response to a person, experience or desire in life.

When we are hurt as a child or younger person, it's not uncommon to respond emotionally in anger with an inner vow to curse something or avoid the source of that pain. If we were whipped by a parent, and it embarrassed us, then it would be an expected response as a child to vow to never whip or discipline our own kids. While that might sound like a noble gesture at the time, the reality is that a parent who refuses to discipline their children will only grow to see unruly kids without structure.

Not to mention, a spouse who may grow frustrated by your refusal to take charge of the kids. Beyond their displeasure at your failing to father the children, and the bad uncorrected behavior of the kids, your spouse's dissatisfaction stems from not understanding why you refuse to correct your very own children.

The truth is, you probably don't remember making that inner vow as a young child while on the receiving end of a switch or belt. But the reality is, once you make these self-directed statements, you have the potential for igniting a pattern of dysfunction and misery.

Other common inner vows are:

- I'll never let anyone hurt me again.
- I'll never be poor like my parents
- I'll never trust anyone again.
- I'll give my own kids everything they want.
- I'll never let my wife talk to me that way.
- I'll never wait on God to do something I want now.

Do these sound familiar? I'll give you a chance to write out your own in a bit, but for now, think through the times you may have purposefully or inadvertently made inner vows out of embarrassment, anger or frustration. The danger is with the self-oriented intention.

Anything directed inward, as opposed to outward or upward to God, eliminates God from the process, and most importantly the outcome. Is accumulating wealth bad? No, God wants to bless us in all things, but when the accumulation was made as a result of an inner vow, then God was not part of the process. This opens the door for money to become your god (lower case g).

Because you were embarrassed by being poor as a child, you now find yourself outside of God's will and blessings just so you could show Him and your family that you are in control. That's a dangerous and painful place to be.

Because we are focusing on freeing ourselves from past personal pain, inner vows not only imprint a pattern of self-reliance, but from the moment of that vow, we're tethered to that moment in the past. The irony is that whatever you promised to escape, flee from or avoid earlier in life, will continue to haunt you because you're chained to it via the inner vow.

Remember when we talked about soul ties? This is right there with shackles to the past. They can and must be broken in order to move forward and free from the effects of pain.

Three of the most dangerous aspects of inner vows are:

1. They Are Unscriptural:

God says do not swear at all (Matthews 5:33-37) because it doesn't submit itself to God. Jesus says "perform your oaths to the Lord..." but with inner vows, there is no obligation or submission to God. Everything done and accomplished is done internally for self-gratification.

OATHS

> *"Again, you have heard that it was said to the people long ago, 'Do not break your oath, but fulfill to the Lord the vows you have made.' But I tell you, do not swear an oath at all: either by heaven, for it is God's throne; or by the earth, for it is his footstool; or by Jerusalem, for it is the city of the Great King. And do not swear by your head, for you cannot make even one hair white or black. All you need to say is simply 'Yes' or 'No'; anything beyond this comes from the evil one.*
> *Matthew 5:33-37*

2. They Have An Unseen Effect:

As we discussed earlier, you may not even realize that you locked your future self into a pattern of behavior outside of God's will. And while it may take years or even decades before you understand what is going down, it eventually comes to a head for conflict.

This is called the "sleeper" effect, and results from a vow lying dormant until triggered by an action or response. When examined through God goggles, you see how much hurt has been suffered by you and caused to others by you. Inner vows create this pain environment because you're in charge and God isn't.

3. They Are The Most Powerful Form Of Commitment:

Inner vows are powerful because they were made by you, and at a time of hurt or turmoil that affected you. Because you personally removed God from the equation, you have a tendency to cling to the vow no matter what the cost to you or others.

Pain, anger and desperation make for a lethal combination. You will not know inner peace until you have freed yourself from the consequences of selfish inner vows.

HOW TO UNLOCK INNER VOWS

The first step to breaking free from the shackles of an inner vow is to identify the vow itself. I know it's impossible to retrace every thought or word spoken over the course of your life. But if you begin by looking back on times that your parents failed you, or at least at the time you thought they failed you, that is a great start.

Next, think through negative events, moments and actions related to life moments. Were there times where you passed strong judgments about your parents, or your past, or about your ideals for your future?

I'll share one from my childhood, and although it seemed innocent, as I matured, it caused grief for me and my family. There were seven kids in my family. My parents rushed us from ball practice to the grocery store as best they could with one car.

The result was a few times arriving late to practice or an event. It drove me nuts and I would complain from the time we left until they dropped me off. I swore I'd never be late once I was able to drive.

For decades, that inner vow caused an obsession with punctuality. Now before you say, that's a good thing, did you catch that I said an "obsession"? That not only went for me, but anyone who worked for me, my wife, kids, friends, people in the drive-thru, airlines, etc.

At the source, it was more about a selfish boy not wanting to miss a single pitch or be embarrassed by sprinting across the field after everyone else had arrived. I also placed harsh judgment against my parents although they hustled more than anyone I knew just so we wouldn't have to miss out on being involved.

While I obsessed over time, I didn't waste any time in rebuking that inner vow and praying freedom and restoration over it. I was amazed, once freed, at how much stress it used to cause in my daily life. Yeah, and everyone else's too.

Inner vows are connected to the level of strong judgments and unforgiveness against people in your life. To break free and liberate yourself from the past pains that prompted the vows, you must identify them, confess them, repent and pray for God's restoration.

Call To Action

1. Write out in detail what you understand to be your inner vows.

2. Write out in detail what you remember as the cause for having prompted you to make the inner vows.

3. Write out periods in your life that you have condemned others with strong judgments that have led to making inner vows.

4. Write out in detail one example of an inner vow and how it affects you today.

9

JUDGMENTS

You, therefore, have no excuse, you who pass judgment on someone else, for at whatever point you judge another, you are condemning yourself, because you who pass judgment do the same things.
Romans 2:1

This is an important section to discuss because God's word covers judgment all throughout the Bible. The effects of passing judgment are rooted in spiritual laws and consequences. I'm sure as you're reading this, your mind has already wandered off to, "judge not, lest ye be judged."

Yeah, so has mine. This is how vital it is to understand the connection between judging and past pain. Without even knowing where that line from the Bible is located, it's indelibly embedded in our brains. It's Matthew 7:1 by the way, but I'll share more of that and other key scripture showing you both sides of the blessing or curse that we rain down upon ourselves with judgments.

Now, let's be honest about making judgment about others. I'm guilty of it, and although I really try avoiding casting judgment upon others, I still catch myself doing it. When we do this, it's similar to placing a curse in action. Except that according to God's word, we reap what we sow, as well as we are judged by the same measure that we have judged.

We live under two very certain and undeniable laws as set forth by God in His creation of this world. The spiritual laws reveal God's character, and the physical laws which govern the world we live in. When we judge others, we set the spiritual laws into effect that, while we may not recognize, are still very much in action.

The law of judgments is critical for us to understand as they apply to attaching ourselves to past pain, and again, like other tethers to our past, these must be dealt with according to scripture. But first, let me show you around the authorization for these actions found throughout God's word, but most specifically in these verses:

1. **Romans 2:1** - *Therefore, every one of you who judges is without excuse. For when you judge another, you condemn yourself, since you, the judge, do the same things.*
2. **Luke 6:37** - *Do not judge, and you will not be judged. Do not condemn, and you will not be condemned. Forgive, and you will be forgiven.*
3. **Matthew 7:1-2** - *Do not judge, so that you won't be judged. For you will be judged by the same standard with which you judge others, and you will be measured by the same measure you use.*

When we judge someone, we are assessing a value, usually a diminished value on that person. Yet, who are we to judge anyone? This is where the violation occurs, and it is not without consequence. God is our king and our judge, so when we do it, we not only remove Him from our life, but we take His place.

In these three scriptural verses we see that by judging another, we are condemned, we are ourselves judged, and we are judged by the same measure or standard we used against the other person.

When I was a kid with six siblings, I loved to fight, mock and tease all of them no matter how much older some were. My mother warned me against making ugly faces at them and said one day that ugly face would stick. Although she didn't realize it, she was right on the mark about violating God's law of judgments. The ugly nature we show others is what we will be shown.

The seeds we sow in our youth or earlier adulthood will always come back to be reaped. It might be an immediate response or lay dormant for decades before rearing its head. But you can be sure that who and what you condemn will become you and what you despise most.

We've covered and will continue to examine the effects of past personal pain and its effects on us today. So much of the pain we carry is a result of our childhood and earlier life. Sometimes that pain results from injury or physical abuse, while other times it occurs when abandoned or neglected. In all of these main instances, pain results from our being a victim.

In the incident of judgment, just as in the case of making inner vows, we are the instigator. A guy whom I never met personally, but we'll call Troy, asked me to mentor him through text and social media. He confessed he struggled with alcoholism. Of course, his drinking led to being fired from several jobs and one divorce. He was deep into the process for his second and wanted desperately to save the marriage.

He was very upfront about the abuse of alcohol to cover feeling bad about himself. He'd thought about suicide, but he said he believed in God and was afraid of the consequences. To me, that was a great sign that Troy was in it to win it, but he just didn't have the tools to get the job done.

We began to discuss his past, and not surprising, he had major conflicts with his dad. His father was a hard worker who hit the bottle as soon as he hit the front door. While neither Troy, nor his mom were physically abused when his dad was drunk, they were neglected. His dad's drinking led to physical ailments and loss of work and then poverty for the family before he walked away from his wife and Troy.

Troy hated his dad for what he'd done to his mom and him. He swore he'd never drink a drop of alcohol and cursed his dad because of it. Troy's bitter judgment of a man who also had an alcoholic, but horribly abusive father (Troy's grandfather), caused Troy to become the object that his judgment hated; a divorced alcoholic.

We worked backward through his past until he was able to identify not only soul ties, but the inner vow based on a condemning judgment against his father. Troy worked to confess his sin, repent and pray for God's restoration with his wife.

Sowing and Reaping

Troy was fortunate to have plugged into God's spiritual laws before he'd again found himself divorced for a second time. His violation is also an example of moving beyond just the law of judgment, and into the spiritual realm of sowing and reaping. Both are closely connected.

Do not be deceived: God cannot be mocked. A man reaps what he sows. Whoever sows to please their flesh, from the flesh will reap destruction; whoever sows to please the Spirit, from the Spirit will reap eternal life. Let us not become weary in doing good, for at the proper time we will reap a harvest if we do not give up.
Galatians 6:7-9

1. Whatever you sow will come back to you.
2. Whatever you sow will multiply upon return.
3. Whatever you sow will be reaped in its own time.
4. Whatever you sow will return in like fashion. Good cannot come from bad, nor will bad come from good seed.

"No good tree bears bad fruit, nor does a bad tree bear good fruit. Each tree is recognized by its own fruit. People do not pick figs from thornbushes, or grapes from briers.
Luke 6:43-44

There is spiritual authority in our words. Our tongue has the power of life and death, so if you sincerely want to gain freedom from your past, please weigh your words wisely. Especially regarding harsh judgments of other people. Speak truth to power and life-giving encouragement to others, and you shall receive blessings of like kind.

Call To Action

1. Write out in detail condemning words of judgment that you commonly speak.

2. Write out in detail three judgments against people in your past.

3. Write out whether what you judged these people for have carried over to characteristics you now exhibit.

4. Write out a prayer confessing your judgment, request for forgiveness and your blessings for those you harmed.

10

UNFORGIVENESS

21Once you were alienated from God and were enemies in your minds because of your evil behavior. 22 But now he has reconciled you by Christ's physical body through death to present you holy in his sight, without blemish and free from accusation— 23 if you continue in your faith, established and firm, and do not move from the hope held out in the gospel. This is the gospel that you heard and that has been proclaimed to every creature under heaven, and of which I, Paul, have become a servant.
Colossians 1:21-23

Our discussions about forgiveness can sometimes get confusing and slide off the rails when we get hung up on "letting their offender off the hook." I feel like we've covered the realities of God's command to forgive, and that the process is about setting you free from your offenders and allowing God to take His vengeance.

Now let's talk about unforgiveness. It's pretty simple. If you do not forgive others, God will not forgive you. I've been known to be pretty hardheaded in my life, but even I understand that.

*But if you do not forgive others their sins,
your Father will not forgive your sins.
Matthew 6:15*

Because God commands us to forgive, the fact that we either can't or won't is a direct attack on God's word. In other words, not forgiving is a sin, and a sin you will not be forgiven for because you've refused or failed to forgive others. Once we place ourselves into an environment of separation from God, there are a ton of adverse effects just waiting to happen.

This isn't the time to go all sad sack and say, "Why me?" The answer isn't that God punishes us; it's that we've removed ourselves from beneath His hedge of protection and opened ourselves to the results of sin.

The solution is so simple. Forgive others as God has told us to do. It's not just so we'll do as He says, but it's a lifesaving and changing experience that draws us closer to the true heart of God's loving compassion. It's also the only way to genuinely change our heart toward others.

There is a negative power found with unforgiveness, and it has the potential to destroy you. Just to show you how serious this business is; God forgives all sin except for one. Blaspheming the Holy Spirit is the single unforgivable, eternal sin.

*Truly I tell you, people can be forgiven all their sins and every slander they utter, but whoever blasphemes against the Holy Spirit will never be forgiven; they are guilty of an eternal sin."
Mark 3:28-29*

But, look back at Matthew 6:15, and see that although sin can be forgiven, it will not be. Now, we're not talking about blaspheming the Holy Spirit, but we are talking about refusing to forgive others. Either way, the outcome of not being forgiven is the same. The difference is, you do have the grace of God's covering, but you chose not to accept His gift.

For the wages of sin is death; but the gift of God is eternal life through Jesus Christ our Lord.
Romans 6:23

And to wrap up this section with some more simple truth, sin brings death. Not automatically a physical death, but a separation from God. And because we do have the blessing of free will, we also have the ability to accept His gift of eternal life as opposed to the alternative. Seems like it's time to start forgiving those who have sinned against you.

I'd like to share a key example of how unforgiveness negatively affects us. Matthew 18:21-35 shares the conversation between Jesus and Peter in which they discuss forgiveness and how often must someone be willing to forgive. When and if we do forgive someone, most of us have the one-and-done attitude. Jesus has a very different number in mind.

Jesus also backed up His command of forgiving someone not seven times, but seventy times seven times. Now, before we write down 490, let's look at the historical reality behind that number. The tradition was that if you forgave someone three times, you were a very good person. Peter's question to Jesus included the traditional three, and he doubled it for good measure and added one to be sure. Seven times forgiven would surely make one a saint, right?

Seemed like everyone was trying to trip up Jesus, even His closest friends. Sounds familiar?

Jesus gives the number seventy times seven not as a hard target, but to show that we never stop forgiving. Forgiving is a never-ending practice of mercy and grace. Just as Christ died for our sins once, His blood covers our sins for eternity. We are to forgive in all occasions and without limit or conditions.

Why? Because unforgiveness causes us pain. It also prevents us from escaping our past that caused the pain. If you were abused by a parent or adult; your refusal to forgive them keeps you shackled to that person and that harmful action. So unforgiveness not only puts us out in the cold from God's presence, but while out there, we're still attached to what hurt us in the first place. Not surprisingly, it's God that we need to set us free, but because we've turned from Him, we don't have the gift of His freedom-giving power.

Getting back on track with the parable Jesus uses in Matthew 18:21-35, He tells about a master who forgave his servant a massive debt as opposed to tossing him in prison and allowing the tormentors to have their way with him. The servant was so thankful, he snatched up a fellow servant who owed him very little. Unable to repay the debt, the original servant who was just forgiven a huge debt, had the fellow servant thrown into prison and tortured.

Not surprising, word got back to the master who had once forgiven his servant. He had the unforgiving servant tossed into prison and also tortured until his insurmountable debt was repaid. The reality was, that guy would never be able to repay his master what he owed. Do you see how this is us when we fail to forgive?

God sacrificed His only begotten Son so that our sins would be forgiven once and for eternity. The example of forgiving is the greatest love sacrifice ever, and something we could never repay God. Yet, when He asks us to forgive one another, we balk because we've been harmed, or our feelings got hurt.

Don't misunderstand the negative power of unforgiving. It does cause pain and can lead to physical illnesses and emotional misery. It's sort of a pain prison where the ones we refuse to forgive are our jailers. They tug the chain, and we feel the pain. We can cut that invisible cord right this second by forgiving them.

Remember the three keys to genuinely forgive someone:

1. Repent – Unforgiveness is a sin, so before forgiving those who have sinned against you, make the time to repent for your own sin of unforgiving.
2. Release – We've talked about judgments against others, and their effect on our own lives. To genuinely forgive, we must break the curse and release the judgment against others.
3. Bless – God is very clear that it's a two-step process. Not

only must we forgive those who have sinned against us, but we must bless them.

I want to wrap this up with a quick story about a guy we'll call Abe. When we began working together, he said the same thing as you might've said after reading number 3 about blessing those who have offended you. All I asked while mentoring him was that he keep his mind and heart open to the Holy Spirit.

He hated his ex-wife, the mother of their one child. Sharing, he said she was a horrible woman who after almost 15 years, still tried to torment and manipulate him. Abe had remarried after being divorced ten years, but that seemed to only set her off even more. She caused Abe stress and it affected his life and his new wife.

Abe and I prayed that God would move him to begin praying forgiveness for his ex-wife. He began speaking it out loud as he drove to work. Although the words choked him at first, he began to feel the burden of the hatred and judgment he carried slip away from him. We celebrated his breakthrough, but then...

I explained that he had to also bless her. He balked. I explained that he had to bless her not just with his mouth but in his heart. Abe's first words were, "I can't do it. She doesn't deserve God's blessings."

I understood his hesitation to bless her. It wasn't a natural inclination to bless those who hurt us. And, that was the point! In our natural posture, we cannot do this, but in our spiritual man, All things are possible through Christ.

I asked Abe if he loved his daughter, who was 9 at the time. Of course, he answered with a very resounding yes. I followed up with wouldn't he want his daughter to live in a home where her mother found Christ and walked in the same spirit of faith as Abe and his wife. He gave another resounding yes.

"Then why are you withholding that blessing from your daughter?" Were the exact words I asked him. Tears shed as Abe's last thin veil of resistance was shredded. He later shared that he had to baby-step the process of blessing his ex-wife each day until his thoughts became embedded in his heart.

Please remember that God dearly loves those whom we may hate.

Call To Action

1. Write out why you either cannot, will not or refuse to forgive others.
2. Write out the names of 3 people who you need to forgive.
3. Write out separately in detail what each person's offenses were.
4. Write out a prayer of forgiveness for each person

11

SOUL SCARS

20For the creation was subjected to frustration, not by its own choice, but by the will of the one who subjected it, in hope 21 that the creation itself will be liberated from its bondage to decay and brought into the freedom and glory of the children of God.
Romans 8:20-21

Injury causes pain. It also causes scars that serve as a reminder of the pain and the injury. Unlike physical healing, emotional, mental and spiritual injuries don't heal over time. While the body launches into an immediate recovery phase after experiencing a wound, your spirit remains vulnerable. As a matter of fact, those injuries get more severe the longer left unattended.

Time does not heal all wounds.

My wife and I were talking about parents and pain one afternoon. So much of our dysfunction can be linked directly to things they did or didn't do during our childhood. I'd remarked that it was almost impossible to be a parent and not mess up your kids.

The truth is, no one is perfect. Through our lives we will hurt and be hurt. The difference for parents who believe in Jesus Christ is that they've place Him as the God head of their marriage and children. Following the Christ example helps parents minimize the damage or recognize it when done and work to restore the child.

The truth to remember is the scars on our spirit will not heal until we allow them to be healed. So, I know you might respond like I first did. Why wouldn't we want to allow ourselves to be healed? Well, to be honest, there are several reasons, but intimidation and being ridiculed by others are the top two.

If you'll recall earlier, I shared an experience of investigating a serial child molester. Although we'd identified and contacted victims going back over twenty years, none of the men would admit they were molested by the man while they were kids. Sure, these men were victims and they needed help in the worst way, but they'd rather exist in their fractured husks, than reclaim victory through Christ.

I'm not, and never would condemn them. It was their choice, and although I grieved for each one's loss of childhood innocence, I understand the personal choices each must make. The point I want to share is that there are many reasons people don't seek healing, and these are just two.

You'd also be surprised to know that in this world of everything online, many of us don't know where to get the help to heal. Where do we begin? Since most of us want to avoid the risk of public exposure, asking others for help or a reference limits potential resources right off the bat.

I will share that there are several levels of care that you may need depending on how deep your injuries go. But, because there is a spiritual connection between cause and cure, I always suggest that people seek out the counsel of their pastor. Many faith leaders are trained and focus their ministry on healing the hurts that harm our walk with Christ.

If you have a pastor, please go speak with him. If it is a situation requiring another level of care, they will refer you. Don't feel as though you are being passed around. Each situation is different and may require care ranging from conversation to medication. But you'll never know unless you're willing to trust someone to get started in the healing process.

If you are suffering and don't think you need to trust opening up to someone, then you're experiencing yet another reason why we remain trapped in pain: denial.

We'll go to just about any length to avoid something we have zero interest or understanding in. One of the most common ways we do this is by suppressing emotions about the event. We can't hurt because we're self-reliant after all, right? The best way to avoid the pain is to avoid the feelings associated with it. That's like saying if I avoid the blood running out of my chest, then the bullet that's in there will go away.

Was that example a little too graphic? Sorry, an occupational hazard of police work. But I hope you get the point. Disassociation is a tactic we use to distance ourselves from the act that hurt us. But even if the distance is actually physical space, the tether that ties you to it is always right around the corner. Besides, you can't selectively shut off one emotion without adversely effecting other emotions.

Destructive behavior such as defensiveness, external influencers like drugs and alcohol, exponentially increase the risk and damage caused by the pain. Bigger problems arise once our focus is now placed on fighting addictions as opposed to healing the wounds that caused the pain requiring us to "medicate" ourselves.

Like most things in life, there is a process involved. So just in case you are curious why God doesn't just snap His fingers and make your pain go away, it's important to understand the different type of healing.

Instant Healing by Miracle:

There are numerous examples of immediate healing performed by God or God through Jesus. They were quick and seemed effortless on behalf of Jesus. Despite the various ailments, the common factor besides Jesus was that those healed believed in the power to be healed.

Healing by Process:

Whether healing is instant or occurs over a long period of time, it is the process for restoration. God may speed it up, or slow it down, but never forget that God sets the pace and the degree of restoration. What is important is that God's word promises the end result, not how long it takes.

How often have we passed through a trial and once it's over, we've either forgotten what we've been through, or came to understand the changes in our lives as a result of having gone through something. Part of God's healing process is education.

Remember when Lazarus's family begged Jesus to run to him? What did Jesus do? He took four days before he arrived at the tomb of his friend. Lazarus had even begun to rot, and his flesh stunk, but Jesus was in no hurry. Why wasn't He?

There was a process. There were people besides Lazarus who would benefit in faith through this process, and while the end result was imminent, the process vetted out doubts, fears and hope from those attached to the process. Read John 11:1-46 for yourself and mark down how many people close to Christ behaved less than faithfully.

Just as in the example of Lazarus being raised from the dead, there were feelings present during the process of healing. Men, no matter how hard we try to pretend we don't have feelings, the truth is we do. Now, it doesn't mean we have to weep at the coffee shop or during halftime of our favorite team, but the process of healing from past personal pain involves our being able to understand why we feel the way we do.

ANGER

Denial bottles up lots of emotion. We don't process those emotions, so they have to find outlets. Once we open up to the process of healing, we'll see that anger has been waiting to rage for a while.

This anger also has two options – to manifest internally or externally. Usually anger is directed at whomever it was that hurt you. If it was your dad, then you may seek out revenge, but please understand the consequences. Restoration is a much better option.

Instead of seeking out the one who caused your pain, some people attack themselves through shame, guilt or depression for allowing themselves to have been victimized. Please don't measure your adult expectations by the child's reactions.

Remember in either outlet, you are not responsible for what was done to you, but you are now responsible for how you handle it. Also, since we're giving good one-liner advice, anger is not a sin, as long as you don't sin in your anger.

> *"Be angry, and do not sin":*
> *do not let the sun go down on your wrath.*
> *Ephesians 4:26*

GRIEVING

Similar to the stages of death and loss, we must process our emotions. Unlike death where there is either no notice or a relatively contained period before the loss, the emotional upheaval we'll have to face has been buried just below our spirit's surface since the injury.

Grieving is important for allowing a balance to anger. It usually begins as the process of anger is resolved or managed. You may feel as though these days are your darkest and you can't hold on any longer but let me assure you that healing is yours.

This is the season Jesus has been waiting for. He sincerely wants to help you, but He will not force Himself into a situation where He is not welcomed. Let's look at Revelation's illustration.

> *Behold, I stand at the door and knock. If anyone hears My voice and opens the door, I will come in to him and dine with him, and he with Me.*
> *Revelation 3:20*

Christ has been waiting on you, but the denial, anger, disassociation and every layer of separation you placed between yourself and the reality of what has harmed you, has created a barrier. Now is the time to tear that wall down between you and the healing grace of Jesus Christ. This is an example of when I mentor men, I tell them from the start that if they do not have a teachable spirit, the relationship will not bear fruit.

ACCEPTANCE

Rarely are we harmed by strangers. What makes the hurt so much more intense is the loss of innocence and trust from the known person. There was an expected honor code of adult protector that was violated.

That violation not only left soul scars because of what action was perpetrated, but that the trust was broken. The physical body can heal itself or be healed. The soul scars are very different, and responses to violations of trust hurt deeper than broken bones or bruises.

Once we have processed our healing and as part of that, been able to forgive and bless those who hurt us, a spirit of acceptance gives us peace. It is not a feeling of joy or happiness, but it is a long-gone peace over what had once hurt you having been processed and placed in the past so you may move forward in the life God created you to enjoy.

Call To Action

1. Write out what you picture your soul scars to be.
2. Write out a list of who caused soul scars upon your spirit.
3. Write out a list of who on the previous list has yet to be forgiven by you.
4. Write out in detail how you have compensated in ways for avoiding having to deal with the pain.
5. Write out a prayer for your coming to heal completely.

12

UNSEEN ENEMIES

Therefore, there is now no condemnation for those who are in Christ Jesus, 2 because through Christ Jesus the law of the Spirit who gives life has set you free from the law of sin and death. 3 For what the law was powerless to do because it was weakened by the flesh, God did by sending his own Son in the likeness of sinful flesh to be a sin offering. And so he condemned sin in the flesh, 4 in order that the righteous requirement of the law might be fully met in us, who do not live according to the flesh but according to the Spirit.
Romans 8:1-4

I truly appreciate you sticking with me throughout this. I've prayed over our work and the effort we're putting into this, and I know it's challenging, but worth it. It has changed my life. One of the things that took a while to understand with clarity is in the realm of unseen enemies.

Of course, we probably all have those people out there who, for whatever reason, do not like us or have a penchant for causing grief. But I'm talking about the spiritual realm, and satanic forces. This is also where some people either flip to the next chapter, or balk at the progress they've made so far and check out. Don't do it; stick together.

Please, hang with me for a bit and I'll show you scriptural evidence that the devil does exist and is wholly invested in separating us from God. My pastor helped me to understand the battle that has raged for thousands of years, but in the beginning, I was unsure of what I was being told.

For our struggle is not against flesh and blood, but against the rulers, against the authorities, against the powers of this dark world and against the spiritual forces of evil in the heavenly realms.
Ephesians 6:12

A man who I love and adore had been invited to serve as one of the chaplains for my police department while I was the chief. He would tell me that my battle wasn't against crime in the city; it was a supernatural war between good and evil. To be honest, it freaked me out a bit at first, and if I had my choice at that moment, I would've stuck to fighting bad guys.

I soon saw what it was he was talking about. He continued to pray over me and petition God to sustain me in that spiritual fight. I'll confess that it got intense at times. As I became more comfortable with accepting the reality of natural and spiritual realms, the Holy Spirit became more valuable to me than all of the cops in my agency.

I'll share a few things I learned during that experience as a leader tasked with mentoring and protecting others.

1. The supernatural realm is very real.
2. This is not a battle we can win on our own.
3. The war has already been won with the crucifixion and resurrection of Jesus Christ.
4. The attacks are relentless, but God has given us His armor of protection.
5. Satan uses anyone and everyone against you. Even yourself.

6. Through faith we have the authority to resist the devil and he will flee.
7. Satan is not God, so he is not omnipresent, but he has legions of demons at his command.
8. There is no neutral ground in this war. You are either under the grace of God or control of Satan.

The pain, shame and guilt you've carried with you is a result of the devil's consistent campaign to keep you separated from God. That's his entire purpose because once he's got you on your own, you're easy prey. The devil specializes in the world of steal, kill and destroy. Once you are divided from God, you'll soon find yourself apart from your wife, kids, life and faith. Everything that is important to you becomes a target for this sharpshooter.

Even the devil's name is rooted in division. *Dia-bolos* in Greek references, "the one who divides." Ever watched those wildlife shows? The predator rushes into the pack to divide them. They spot the weaker animals, so they launch toward them again. They divide the smaller group to flee the predator. Finally, you may see the vulnerable one with one other animal, usually the mother of the intended victim. But, skilled as the predator is, the last approach divides even them and leaves the target alone and defenseless.

We just talked about the need for Christ to begin healing the soul scars from our past. It's impossible without Him. This is why it's so crucial for Satan to divide us from God so that we remain in our pain and sin. In that state, there is no healing, only continued pain.

While we're better off focusing on the miraculous authority of God's dominion over this world than Satan's efforts to destroy it, I wanted to give a few scriptural references to verify the demonic presence on this earth. It's really too bad people, even believers, have minimized Satan into a rogue with horns and a pointy tail. He is much more than a cartoon.

Be alert and of sober mind. Your enemy the devil prowls around like a roaring lion looking for someone to devour.
1 Peter 5:8

In Revelation, Jesus states very clearly that the devil, and a third of the angels who followed him were not only cast out of heaven, but specifically throw to earth.

The great dragon was hurled down—that ancient serpent called the devil, or Satan, who leads the whole world astray. He was hurled to the earth, and his angels with him.
Revelation 12:9

Since the devil made his first appearance in the Garden of Eden, he's been on the prowl for you and me. There are four primary tactics used by the devil to interfere in our walk with Christ.

1. *Deception* – This is his master skill set. He manipulates us into thinking we are broken and beyond or unworthy of healing. Satan leads us to believe God doesn't love us, so we don't deserve to be healed. He's the father of lies, so anything negative you think of to stop you from breaking free from past personal pain is the work of the devil.
2. *Occult Activity* – God warned us about witchcraft, but for some rebellious reason, His people have been vulnerable to activities, music, movies, rituals and anything Satan deceives them into believing holds special power. God holds the power, not tricks and charms.
3. *Physical Illness* – While Satan is not a god, he does rule over a kingdom. Within his kingdom are legions of demons at various ranks such as any established army. Demonic possession is real, and God's word gives us numerous examples of physical healings once spirits were cast out.

1. *Mental Disorders* – Not every form of mental disorder is demonic, but beyond health defect, many are. Even the effects of low self-esteem, fear, shame, insecurity and depression can be linked to the devil's lies and division. He causes doubt which leads to separation from God.

Let's wrap up this with the good news of Jesus Christ. A very big part of His ministry's emphasis was on healing and deliverance. Jesus cast out demons to restore health and stability. He still heals, and He will heal you by setting you free from the bonds of your past pain. But you must allow Him in.

Call To Action

1. Write out all personal experiences of demonic interference in your faith walk with Christ.

2. Write out where you see yourself in the supernatural battle within the spiritual realm.

3. Write out a battle plan to prevent Satan from invading your life. Maybe he enters through alcoholism, abuse, porn, or some sin-based addiction or behavior that creates an open door for his indwelling.

13

SPIRITUAL OPPRESSION

This matter arose because some false believers had infiltrated our ranks to spy on the freedom we have in Christ Jesus and to make us slaves.
Galatians 2:4

While preparing to write a book based on scripture, educational resources and personal experiences, I always loosely organize the materials and then hand it over to the Holy Spirit to sort it out. Better than any editor, the Holy Spirit is concise in what should and shouldn't be in each section. It's a discipline of submission, and one that I'm continuing to pursue.

The last content that focused on unseen enemies was hard to write. It became a practical application effort as my distraction level caused several days of delay. The Holy Spirit was definitely in my corner as I pushed through doubts and worries about how you might perceive so much focus on the reality of demonic interference in our lives. But, in typical Holy Spirit fashion, there was no option than to present the truth.

When I felt I'd come to the end of the topic, I soon felt that familiar tug. There was more about demonic, spiritual oppression to share. I know we get uncomfortable talking about the spiritual realm. It's outside of things we can grab onto and rattle or finesse until fixed. But it plays a huge role in our lives of past personal pain.

While not biblical, I thought about Sun Tzu's quote, and I paraphrase, "Know thy enemy, know thyself." This is true for people who are struggling against something beyond themselves, a family member, co-worker, or others.

Let's not play games here; the enemy is the devil and he is out to kill, steal and destroy. God's word describes him as a lion looking to devour you. So, it is important to know the enemy. Actually, our lives depend upon it.

For we wrestle not against flesh and blood, but against principalities, against powers, against the rulers of the darkness of this world, against spiritual wickedness in high places.
Ephesians 6:12

I'll confess that the reality of a demonic spirit fighting for space in my life can be a bit intimidating, but that is the truth and if you believe in God, Jesus and the Holy Spirit, then you must accept that they do exist. God says so.

A common concern about demonic possession, is how it affects your life and whether people can actually be possessed. I know most people imagine Linda Blair in *The Exorcist*, but this is real life and a real concern. Discussing the demonic realm is also what stops people from reaching the truth because there's a fear that if we mention it, it might come and get us.

Lack of knowledge creates a boogeyman conception of a very real part of our lives. To answer the question about possession, a Christian cannot be possessed by the devil or a demonic spirit. We were bought by and belong to God. He's doesn't trade us off like a used car for better models. Nonbelievers are a different story. I'd mentioned it before and worth another reminder that if you don't believe and belong to God, then you serve Satan. There is no neutral or middle ground.

> *You were bought at a price. Therefore, honor God with your bodies.*
> *1 Corinthians 6:20*

Possession is one key factor, but there are instances of interference. The best example is if you were a large landowner with title and deed to your property. All because you own the Ponderosa doesn't mean that others won't try squatting on your land. Many settlers in the West discovered unauthorized villages established on their ranches. Without searching your soul, you too may have demonic encampments in your life.

King David went to God himself to search for sin or anything else that would hinder his pursuit of knowing his Father. It's like a virus scan for our computers. Demonic spirits may not be obvious to you, but God is very aware of them, and will wait on you to call out in His name to remove them.

> *Search me, God, and know my heart;*
> *test me and know my anxious thoughts.*
> *See if there is any offensive way in me,*
> *and lead me in the way everlasting.*
> *Psalm 139:23-24*

Demons are not as powerful as Satan, and simply in no comparison to Jesus. Biblical accounts of demonic possession show that they had limited power to only affect a certain part of the inhabitant. Or, in the case of the possessed man at Gerasenes, it required a legion, or 6,000 demons to subdue him.

So, like I said above, while a Christian cannot be possessed by demonic spirits, they can experience limited spiritual suppression. Let's go over the four types, and also how we, as believers open ourselves up to the "squatting" of demons.

1. **Suppression** – This is a low-level interference that is usually in the form of a bad mood. Have you ever been aggravated with your wife or kids but couldn't understand why? You just were. This is usually the case of suppression, and while it's not severe, it can last if not addressed until it becomes a chronic condition.
2. **Mild Oppression** – This level of demonic influence includes deeper and longer lasting bouts with negative moods and emotions. You may struggle to keep your cool, but the effects won't just shake off. For example, if you're fighting with a spirit of anger, you might find yourself going off on people for no reason until you pray over this and rebuke the spirit.
3. **Severe Oppression** – This level is a step beyond mild, and usually involves more than one demon unlawfully staking claim to your spirit. You are now in a real battle for self-control, and often will look back at your behavior and wonder if someone else was running your body. Because of its increased effect, you should also ask other believers to stand with you.
4. **Possession** – This level is not a possibility for Christians. We belong 100% to God, so while we may fight lower level demonic influences, only those who have not been bought by the blood of Jesus Christ are susceptible to true possession. This is a very dangerous situation and requires focused prayer and preparation before confronting.

Now just to be clear, not every bad behavior is of the devil or his demons. We can't rely on the old adage "The devil made me do it," but we have to take this seriously. The devil's the master at deception, so for us to balk at the reality and blow it off as something minor is exactly the Trojan horse he's looking for.

So just how do we find ourselves afflicted with demonic suppression? Demons can't just jump on us. It's not contagious like catching a cold, but there are open access doors that allow them to squat on God's property until expelled.

1. **Sin** – Left unrepentant, sin becomes a superhighway for demonic access.
2. **Unforgiveness** – We've talked about this before, and that if you do not forgive those who sinned against you, God will not forgive you of your sins. This also brings to mind Matthew 18:34's parable where not only are we not forgiven, but we will be handed over to the tormentors until we repay what is due. The bad news is, we cannot ever repay God for what He has given us. So, unless we want to live a life of demonic tormenting, forgiving is not an option.
3. **Parental Sins** – These cast generational curses to the third and fourth generation for families that do not accept Jesus Christ as their savior. Legacy sins also open the door to deep past, personal pain as well as demonic influence. Forgive your parents, whether they are alive or have passed, and take authority for your spiritual life and legacy.
4. **Chemical Addiction** – Drug abuse is a complex situation but is one where opening access to demonic influence is common. Addiction is often the result of struggling to numb past pain through drugs without focusing on the spiritual healing of their pain. This is also an ample access point for demonic activity.
5. **Occult** – I think this goes without needing an explanation. Play with fire, and you're going to get burned.
6. **Physical and Emotional Trauma** – Injury to the body or mind leaves us in a weakened condition. Medications to help the healing process can also introduce us to an altered consciousness. Being aware that you not only have to address the trauma, but the demonic attacks is a great reason to have others stand with you in prayer.

I wanted to cover some of the basic, but most vulnerable attack points of the enemy. The best way to avoid this is by inviting the Holy Spirit in for a constant inventory check.

Let's also remember that not any one of us has the power or authority over the enemy. Only Jesus holds dominion over Satan and his kingdom. Through the authority Jesus invested in Believers, we are commission to resist the devil and his demons. The two requirements for us to resist and cast out demonic influence is that we must be a believer and we must use the name of Jesus Christ.

> *The seventy-two returned with joy and said, "Lord, even the demons submit to us in your name."*
> *He replied, "I saw Satan fall like lightning from heaven. I have given you authority to trample on snakes and scorpions and to overcome all the power of the enemy; nothing will harm you. However, do not rejoice that the spirits submit to you, but rejoice that your names are written in heaven."*
> Luke 10:17-20

Spiritual oppression is real, but God's salvation is eternal.

Call To Action

1. Write out in detail which of the access areas you're most prone to for allowing demons into your life.

2. Write out in detail which types of demonic influence you have experienced.

3. Write out in detail who you still have left to forgive. This one item will change your life.

14

BAGGAGE

The Spirit of the Sovereign LORD is on me, because the LORD has anointed me to proclaim good news to the poor. He has sent me to bind up the brokenhearted, to proclaim freedom for the captives and release from darkness for the prisoners.
Isaiah 61:1

I want to take a moment to share a little of my life, and the experiences that brought me to this point. We've already covered so much, so it's a good time to pump the brakes and reconnect on a more personal level. It's easy to get caught up in the fantasy that the person writing the material must have it all together. Otherwise, how could they write the book?

Personally, I'm a little wary of a coach who never played the game, a healing mentor who's never been hurt, or a Christian who never sinned. I'll assure you I've played the game, been terribly hurt and I've sinned. Thanks be to God, I'm forgiven, I'm healed and I'm a victor in Christ.

So, how did I get to the point of writing this book? God called me into service. Well, He didn't exactly tell me to write a book. But He did place a burden on my heart that was so strong, I left my job to pursue His calling. That calling led to Brick Breakers Men's Ministry and writing this book.

Now to get back on track, when I first met my wife, I carried my suitcase (metaphorical) with pride. It was a high-speed, low weight carbon fiber suitcase with shiny wheels that spun like slick glass. I'd adorned the apparatus with big, bold stickers that told the world and her of my worldly accomplishments.

There was no need to reveal anything to her. Everything I wanted her to know was plastered on the outside of that magnificent suitcase. My favorite stickers read Dad, Police Chief, PhD, Master's Degree, Published Author, College Professor, Triathlete and Single.

They were what defined me and identified who I wanted her and the world to see me as. It was brilliant. I pulled it off without ever having to tug once on that zipper tab. It had to be who I really was if that's how she and others saw me. Right?

We married within the year and looked like we'd perfected the game of husband and wife. It was so simple because she too, had a beautiful, shiny suitcase full of wonderful stickers.

After about a year a strange odor seeped out from my gorgeous suitcase. But the cause had to be something or someone else. Just to be safe, I kept the zipper tab snugged tight against the edge, so nothing got in or out. It was nice and dark inside that case, but it was okay because it had been sealed for decades. And it was beautiful on the outside.

Soon, that odor erupted into a full-blown toxic waste emergency as my once beautiful suitcase of accomplishments was ripped wide open. Inside the secured darkness was a lifetime of pain, shame and regret. There was nothing those once dominant external stickers could do to hold it together. It immediately affected my wife, and I was shocked to see the amount of junk stored inside.

There were a few options available.

If I scrambled to get as much junk as possible back inside, then maybe I could've left her with what I salvaged, and possibly start over with someone unaware of what was back inside that suitcase. Or, if I left it open to air out and allow the bright light of Christ to eradicate the darkness, and begin to heal the junk, then she and I could move forward together.

Two options not available were to pretend it didn't happen or continue in the exposure of a sin-filled life of past pain while she and I kept playing married. Never would either of these be realistic options.

Transparency and accountability became cornerstones to my healing and recovery from a life of dysfunctional living. The irony of that magnificent suitcase was that it was actually baggage. The stickers were earthly accomplishments that were sought out primarily to ease the pain I was never able to escape.

It wasn't until I began to heal that I understood that, instead of my identity being rooted in what I'd accomplished, it should've been grounded in Christ. Did you notice in the earlier list of external stickers, not one of them read, Christian, Believer, Child of God?

That's one of the many things pain does to you. And because the devil is involved in dividing you from your best relationship with Christ, he makes sure you avoid a foundational identity in Christ.

Truth be told; I knew the junk inside that suitcase. I also knew it stunk, because it was my life. But I'd become skilled at keeping it zipped tight and hiding what was ailing me because I'm a man and we cannot show weakness, can we?

I believe we're all strolling around with a similarly awesome suitcase decorated with the stickers we only want others to see. It's totally understandable that we don't want to air our dirty laundry to the world. But when that world gets defined, and the compartment for our loved ones gets really tiny, it's time to consider unzipping that bag and allowing the truth to come out.

You recall the three things I said I would be wary about? Well, let's add a fourth one. I'd be wary about anyone who claims their suitcase contains no baggage. I mean, seriously, unless you've not started kindergarten yet, you've got baggage. Sometimes sharing yours allows them to unpack theirs. Which, by the way, is why I've written this book.

Call To Action

1. Write out in detail what your stickers say about how you identify.

2. Write out in detail what those stickers should actually say to describe you.

3. Write out a laundry list of stinky junk still in your baggage.

4. Write out in detail your commitment to clean that dirty laundry.

15

HOW TO REMAIN SPIRITUALLY FREE

I will walk about in freedom, for I have sought out your precepts.
Psalm 119:45

I've gotten to points in my life where my foot smashed into the floor as a fist beat against the air and I proclaimed, "No more." The day of my declaration, I'd muscle through whatever it was I was going to stop, start or change in my life. I was strong and committed; no problem.

The next day was the problem. Without a plan, I was lost in what to do and what to avoid. My natural inclinations would resurface, and just like that, I was wondering what had happened as I wallowed back into the behavior I'd just committed to stop.

Working for spiritual freedom is so important, but it's like anything from dieting to exercise; without a plan, failure is almost certain. I want to talk about several tactical ideas for helping you stay on the path. Like late night snacks, we can just as easily fall back into the pain pool that has plagued us for years.

Let's start with the continual act of surrender. Some guys see it as a contradiction of terms when we discuss freedom and surrender. We don't see how there can be freedom when giving up is usually associated with captivity. But we're talking about the spiritual realm of freedom and surrender.

SURRENDER

Surrender is not a word we easily embrace. To most of us, it means defeat, failure, overcome, or one of many negative words that offend us. While putting up a valiant effort and resisting the enemy is encouraged, surrendering our lives to Jesus Christ is the victory.

The act of surrendering to God is an act of love and trust. Sacrificial love is the highest expression there is. God gave up His one and only beloved Son so that we may know everlasting life through salvation. We are asked to sacrifice our sinful, selfish desires to God so that He may guide us to a relationship with Him and others.

Why doesn't God just *make* us listen and obey Him, you might ask? That's a great question. God loves us so dearly that he gave us free will. This is what separates us from the animals. Unfortunately, free will is also what's caused nearly all of our troubles beginning with Adam and Eve.

Just to take a step back into history, consider our very first couple ever created. Adam and Eve had it made. They literally lived in paradise and hung out with God every day. Yet, they were given the grace to make their own decisions. God asked them not to eat from the fruit of the tree of knowledge of good and evil, and warned that if they did, they would surely die.

That's sounds pretty simple to me, but they had every right to make their own choices despite the close relationship with God the Father. Guess what? They took a chance, and it caused them and us an eternal separation from God. This is why Jesus came to us as the final atonement for the sin of man.

So, back to the point, God will not make us do anything. This is why surrender is the ultimate act of love for God. Now, once we humble ourselves to a position of surrender, we may come to know truth through Christ. Through that truth comes spiritual freedom.

You will know the truth, and the truth will set you free!"
John 8:32

Please don't carry that old resistance to the term surrender or submit. These are terms of ultimate, sacrificial love as God exhibits it. Before you may know spiritual freedom from your past, you must gain a current understanding of freedom's truth. That truth will only come when you put down your weapons of resistance and give your life to Christ. This act of loving surrender will also help you to maintain your well-earned spiritual freedom.

SOUL TIES

We've talked about soul ties earlier, but they are so vital to us gaining and maintaining true freedom from our past pain, that I'd like to revisit it while we discuss spiritual freedom.

Soul ties also continue to play a role in your ability to separate yourself from the injuries caused in your past. Whether the past was decades or days ago, you must gain victory over anything that has pierced your spirit to leave a lasting stain.

We get tethered to people, events, reminiscences (true or false) and feelings from our past. There's a difference between memories and soul ties. Memories are recollections of the past that stir a memory. Soul ties are tangible attachments to the past that can create dysfunction in your present.

It's important for your freedom to spend the time to identify these tethers and release yourself from them through confession, forgiveness and restoration through Christ. New ones develop while old ones may return if we fail to maintain our walk with Christ.

DAILY PRAYER

Talking about our daily walk with Christ, the best way to pursue that relationship is through daily prayer. Whether it's our wife, kids, friends or work, little to nothing gets done without communication. How often does God want to connect with us? His word makes it very clear.

Pray without ceasing
1 Thessalonians 5:17

God wants to share a close relationship with us. I know, it sometimes blows my mind that the creator of everything actually wants to hang out with me.

King David, who God loved so dearly, often struggled with the bigness of God wanting to know him. But the truth is, we were created to glorify Him, and relationships are the best way to do this.

Then King David went in and sat before the Lord, and he said: "Who am I, Sovereign Lord, and what is my family, that you have brought me this far? And as if this were not enough in your sight, Sovereign Lord, you have also spoken about the future of the house of your servant—and this decree, Sovereign Lord, is for a mere human![c]
2 Samuel 7:18-19

RETRAIN YOUR BRAIN

There are other tactics to focus on for making sure you maintain spiritual freedom from your personal past pain. Daily prayer is the foundation, in that it helps you to avoid past habits. I hear it all the time that we cannot control what pops into our mind. I want to assure you that you can. If we look at the brain as an open, unattended back door, then yes, of course sinful thoughts filled with temptation are going to invade your mind and spirit.

God gifted you with an incredible computer, and it's yours to control. What you feed your mind is what your mind will feed upon. The term, "Thoughts that fire together, wire together," is the perfect description of what happens in the programing of your brain.

I've heard the doubters here too, and I only want to assure you that you do have the authority to retrain your brain. It's called neuroplasticity. I like using this example to explain it.

Let's say you're fighting a porn addiction that began as a result of past pain. I want to reassure you that you have the spiritual ability to end that lust for pornography. To begin with, you were not spiritually created with a thirst for porn. God created us to seek one-on-one relationships with each other. Look to Genesis for the creation story of Adam and Eve.

This is why a man leaves his father and his mother and clings to his wife; and they become one flesh.
Genesis 2:24

Adam clung to her and they became one flesh. That becoming one flesh includes their spiritual relationship, but also their physical, sexual combining into one. It is personal, not anonymous relationships that we were designed to pursue.

Next, you were not genetically wired to desire watching porn. As a baby, then toddler, and child and up until you were first exposed to porn, your brain wasn't seeking sex over cartoons. No, it was an exposure to porn that planted a seed of curiosity that grew into an unhealthy dependence for easing your hurts.

Does everyone exposed to porn develop an addiction to it? No, but those who have a spiritual deficit because of pain in our lives are much more prone to it. Just as your brain was exposed to porn and because it was fed a steady diet of it, you can retrain your brain with a steady diet of scripture, prayer and communication with God.

This doesn't only apply to pornography. We must reprogram our minds against all forms of unhealthy, sin-filled thoughts. We can maintain a safe distance from the past that has plagued us, but it requires us to put away the negative sin thoughts. There is good in

God's word, and in this life, but we must pursue it. These are the things God wants us to feed our mind, spirit and soul with.

Finally, brothers, whatever is true, whatever is honorable, whatever is just, whatever is pure, whatever is lovely, whatever is commendable, if there is any excellence, if there is anything worthy of praise, think about these things.
Philippians 4:8

You can do this if you are sincere, purposeful and expectant. You won't just stumble into a command of your thoughts. It can be done if you are committed to making it happen. Look at what the apostle Paul says about our thoughts. He doesn't say smash them if they pop up in your head like a spiritual game of whack-a-mole. He says take them captive and make it obedient.

The words Take and Make are powerful action terms. You are a fixer and a doer, so be that person of action and put these two commands into action in your life.

We demolish arguments and every pretension that sets itself up against the knowledge of God, and we take captive every thought to make it Obedient to Christ.
2 Corinthians 10:5

Call To Action

1. Write out a recurring negative thought in detail.
2. Write out why you think that thought is so dominant in your mind.
3. Write out a creative, imaginative description of a jailer taking that negative thought as a prisoner and subjecting it to the spiritual justice system.
4. Write out three positive memories in detail.

16

DISTORTED IMAGE OF GOD

"The Spirit of the Lord is on me, because he has anointed me to proclaim good news to the poor. He has sent me to proclaim freedom for the prisoners and recovery of sight for the blind, to set the oppressed free.
Luke 4:18

If I were a betting man, I'd say this touches home for most of us. Having a distorted image of God has led us away from Him, or at least caused us to keep God at an arm's length. The way we see God is linked to our willingness to come to him for healing from our past pain.

God created family as a reflection of the way His most immediate family shares in a relationship. The Father, Son and Holy Spirit are each separate but the same because of the seamless love shared. Each lift up and encourages the other with a definite hierarchy with God the Father as the head, Jesus serving His Father, and the Holy Spirit carrying on Jesus's teachings of the Father.

Earthly families were also designed by God for the parents to teach, nurture and encourage their kids. It is because of the intended intimacy shared between parents and the child, that their first understanding of God the Father is engrained at an early age. This is particularly true of the dad, as he on earth serves as the head of the household and is also called father among his children.

Unfortunately, a negative relationship with our dads has the high potential for causing a distorted, and negative perception of God. The reality and most common scenario is that we didn't even understand there was a dysfunctional relationship with our dads. We may never come to know that the way we were treated as kids wasn't what God had intended a parent to show us.

But, it's never too late to come into alignment of a right relationship with God the Father. There is a direct parallel between the image of our parents and God. Once we accept that our parents' behavior does not define the nature of God, we've begun to claim a future of freedom from our past.

I'll share from my own experience. It wasn't until right before turning 50 years old that I came to understand the dysfunctional environment I was raised in. My folks remained married until my mother's death preceded my dad's by about 18 years. So, growing up, I had both parents in the home, yet my dad never spoke with me, said anything nice or said he loved me.

I created an excuse that he was the strong, silent type who showed his love instead of speaking it. I guess if dropping me off to ball practice was showing love, then yes, he loved me. But he never mentored or taught me even the basics of life.

Besides his silence, we never once stepped foot in a church. So, there was nothing to show me otherwise that God the Father was a present, loving God. While I knew there was a God, my perception of Him was of some big, distant guy waiting to whack me when I messed up. Because of that, I found it best to do as I did with my dad by avoiding Him.

When I came to understand that God the Father wasn't like the silent disciplinarian I grew up with, I had to accept that my dad was to be forgiven, blessed and honored.

Captive No More

*"Honor your father and your mother, so that you may live long in the land
the Lord your
God is giving you.
Exodus 20:12*

Without an accurate perception of God, we can't gain true freedom from our past. It's God that sets and keeps us free, so if we still only see Him in the way our parents caused us to view Him, then the seamless relationship needed to act as a rope and a bridge isn't possible.

There are seven attributes of the nature of God that we must see so that there is no doubt that despite our earlier experiences, God is not defined by anyone on this earth. It's an easy trap to remain snared in because dealing with other people is a tangible occurrence as opposed to the spiritual nature of God.

1. God is holy – Holy means that He is separated from sin. Because He is perfect, He cannot look upon us in favor while we carry around unforgiven sin. To draw closer to God, pursue a life of avoiding sin and forgiveness from sin.
2. God is loving and compassionate – The "bigness" of God causes some to see Him as all business without the capacity to love. It is the completely opposite as God is love, and shows mercy, forgiveness and compassion like no human ever could.
3. God is unchangeable – While we've experienced changes in our parents with age or circumstance, the one constant in this existence is God. He is the same God who created Adam and Eve, and the same one who waits with loving patience for you to accept Him. He is the Rock.
4. God is omnipotent – No matter how awesome we might see someone; they are completely limited in their ability. God on the other hand knows no limit. There is nothing He cannot do. God holds authority over the devil, sin, man

and nature. It's sometimes hard for us to comprehend this because His authority is unlimited.
5. God is omnipresent – We find ourselves in some dark places where the empty loneliness seems unrelenting and hopeless. There is nowhere on this planet or the spiritual realm that God is not present. Friend, know that in our worst moments, God is there. All you have to do is call out to Him.
6. God is omniscient – Think of the smartest person in history, or the most talent scientist or even the best game show contestant. The wealth of knowledge, understanding and creativity is infinitesimal compared to the all-knowing nature of God. He knows the number of hairs on your head and the deepest need of your heart. Just open it up to Him.
7. God is faithful – When God starts a work in you, there is no doubt that it will be seen through until the end. How the end looks is often up to us, but God is faithful. His covenants are eternal and unbreakable. He will never leave you or forsake you, and He is the only completely reliable friend you will ever know.

Whether it was your parents, someone else or you that created the distorted image of God, it's now your responsibility to draw into an accurate understanding so that you, too, will know the lasting freedom from your past of personal pain.

Call To Action

1. Write out in detail your first recollection of God.

2. Write out in detail your understanding of God as a child.

3. Write out in detail who most influenced your image of God (good or bad)

4. Write out in detail the nature of your relationship with your parents and how they influenced the way you saw God.

17

DISTORTED SELF-IMAGE

"But whoever listens to me will dwell secure and will be at ease, without dread of disaster."
Proverbs 1:33

Discussing distorted self-images is a super complex topic. I'm not even going to try pigeonholing each of us into some theoretical category. Instead, let's talk about the common issues we face, and how they prevent us from gaining freedom from our past.

I'll start off by confessing that this section really hit home. I saw myself in so many of these scenarios. Or should I say I used to see these situations in my life, but thanks to shattering the shackles of my past pain, I've been set free.

Let's begin by discussing something I know we all struggle with. Guilt, which is a response to something we have done, is not a bad thing to experience. Lacking in or having no guilt is akin to sociopathy, and that's a very bad deal.

Guilt is like cholesterol. There's the good kind that produces conviction, and the bad kind that creates condemnation. Our ability to begin the healing process requires that we embrace one as a compass for change, while avoiding the other as a detour to further complications.

Conviction is a healthy response to the guilt we feel when we sin. It's because we are convicted of wrongdoing, that we seek a path for redemption and restoration. This path is found through confession, repentance, forgiveness and renewal. Let me give a simple run down to show the process:

1. Confession – Confessing our sins shows we are aware of the transgressions, accept the consequences of our actions, and take a posture of accountability and transparency so that God is able to work in our lives.
2. Repentance – is an active term that involves turning away from sin, and having your mind changed about the nature of the activity that involved the sin.
3. Forgiveness – We've talked about this at great length, but if you are the sinner, then we must seek forgiveness from the victim and God. God cannot look upon sin, and without you pursuing forgiveness, He cannot look upon you.
4. Renewal – In Christ we are all new creations. Conviction launches a renewing process so we continue to grow in our Christian faith. We sin; feel guilty about it and are convicted by the Holy Spirit; so, we confess, repent and pursue forgiveness which all brings us into a position of no longer desiring to commit the same sin-filled act. Thus, we are renewed (evolved) into a believer who is more faithful and draws closer to God's will.

On the other side of the guilt coin is condemnation. This leads to nothing helpful for gaining an understanding of what and why we did what we did was wrong, and that through Christ, we are forgiven. All this does is make us feel like failures.

Captive No More

Therefore, there is now no condemnation for those who are in Christ Jesus
Romans 8:1

Shame, although closely related, is not the same as above. While the others are a response to something done, shame is a response to who we are or perceive ourselves to be. You don't focus on what you've done as wrong, but you center your life on a premise that you are bad. Or in my case, I called myself broken for years.

The feelings of shame have no cure through conviction, confession and redemption. It's a label of self-hate that's not easily diminished. You don't just get over being shamed of who you are.

A friend of mine was called to preach years ago. Yes, he'd lived a pretty rough life, and the reason we'd initially met was because I'd arrested him more than a few times. He confided that he first heard the call to serve God but failed to surrender to God's will. Why? Because he was so ashamed of his criminal past.

To be honest, it sort of shocked me. I saw the sweet, genuine spirit nature of the man, but I couldn't get over the criminal man. Unfortunately, neither could he. He never pursued the call to preach, although he maintained a giving life of a sacrificial servant.

Shame is a powerfully destructive force that cannot be ignored or avoided. It can be your Goliath, which means it can be your victory, if you allow God to lead you into the field of battle. It may sound a little cheerleadery, but you must power through the feelings of shame. It was designed to drag you down but has no power to stop you.

Seeing yourself as defective is the height of a distorted self-image. It'll serve as a brick wall in your progress toward freeing yourself from your past. Additionally, shame-bound people may also experience:

1. Denial – often associated with self-deception, and pain avoidance.
2. Obsessive performance – used to manage or avoid feelings of shame. Everything in life becomes a test of your worth,

and the potential or reality of failure is enough to push toward suicide rather than face failure.
3. Striving for Perfection – Control and controlling others is common behavior for the goal for perfection. This is an unhealthy pursuit of the impossible, yet the perfectionist subjects' others to their harsh expectations.
4. Addictions – Hurting people who avoid or deny they are struggling, often turn to ways of numbing the pain. Food, sex, alcohol, drugs are but a few of the "medications" we cling to for relief. Obviously, there is no relief without healing.

I want to also share a condition that we often struggle with as a result of pain, and shame. Relationships are a tool we use to deal with the hurt. As a result of our dysfunctional childhood or family lives, we want to be loved and accepted. Except that we don't want to be accepted for who we are, but who we portray ourselves to be, thanks to self-denial.

But, because we lack the skills to maintain a deep, emotional relationship, they end often. Instead of dealing and healing, we move on to the next attempt at love. Of course, after a pattern of failures, we feel even more shame, and learn to avoid the deep emotions required for a healthy, adult relationship. Shame-bound people are desperate for intimacy, but fail to create the environment for attracting, fostering and keeping it.

The path to healing from the shame that haunts us, requires us to develop four specific behaviors.

1. Recognition – Before we can heal, we must see that there is a problem. Pride and fear interfere with accepting the fact that there is a problem.
2. Determination – Requires repentance and a desire to turn away from sin and destructive practices.
3. Thought-life – One of my favorite sayings is by Albert Einstein: "We can't solve problems by using the same kind

of thinking we used when we created them." We must change our way of thinking. You can reprogram your brain through a process called neuroplasticity.
4. Forgiveness – We've talked about this often, and there's a good reason why. God demands it. If not, the consequences are far too dangerous to risk living outside of God's will.

We were created for relationships. People in pain usually reject intimacy although we suffer more without it. While we may decide to wait until we're healed before making connections, the opposite is true in that until we open up and allow ourselves to connect with others in a healthy, adult relationship, we will never know healing and freedom.

I'm not talking about a new girlfriend or wife. These can be relationships restored by God that were once unhealthy connections, or He can provide for new, fresh fellowship into your life. Either way, it's critical that we change the way we see ourselves and our interactions with others. Freedom comes through healing, and healing comes through intimacy.

Call To Action

1. Write out 10 words that best describe you.

2. Write out why you feel each of these words holds power in your life.

3. Write out Yes or No beside each of the 10 words if that's a word your loved ones would use to describe you.

4. Write out in detail what happened in your last romantic relationship, and why you feel it turned out the way it did – Good or Bad.

18

WRONG RELATIONSHIPS

"For you did not receive the spirit of slavery to fall back into fear, but you have received the Spirit of adoption as sons, by whom we cry, 'Abba! Father!'"
Romans 8:15

We were made for relationships. Now, if you're happily married, you'll probably agree. If you're not happily married, or if you're single, you may wonder what in the world am I talking about and why would I make such a statement. I'll show you through God's word why we were created and that in the creation, relationships were the cornerstone for living a life free from personal pain.

Relationships affect everyone whether we're surrounded by friends and family or locked up in a maximum-security prison cell. We are the way we are today because of the way we were brought up in the context of relationship.

Before humanity existed, God's relational trinity got together and decided to create man in their image. Did you see that? Their image.

Talk about a close relationship, God the Father, Son and Holy Spirit were and still are three in one, the holy trinity.

Then God said, "<u>Let us</u> make mankind in <u>our image</u>, in our likeness, so that they may rule over the fish in the sea and the birds in the sky, over the livestock and all the wild animals, and over all the creatures that move along the ground."
Genesis 1:26

This is important because it's the perfect model, and the beginning of understanding why we were created in the first place. We were created for relationship. When this is out of alignment with God's plan, it causes dysfunction and personal pain for us.

Everyone who is called by my name, whom I created for my glory, whom I formed and made."
Isaiah 43:7

After God created Adam, they shared a loving, intimate relationship. They hung out together and were maybe the first workout partners who walked together daily. Now, despite being in a position of such honor as God's plus-one, Adam wasn't complete. God knew he wasn't meant to alone, so He created his helpmate, Eve.

Here is the beginning of human relationship. The connection with God is the first and most important, and with other humans is next. These are the two most important functions for man. Catching a touchdown pass or getting promoted to executive vice president aren't even close on the scale of what's most important, yet I know we spend more time on those than building the same type of connections as Adam once had with God.

I'll share one more nugget of confirmation about what's our purpose in life. Jesus emphasized the relationship need and hierarchy in Matthew 22:37-40:

Jesus replied: "'Love the Lord your God with all your heart and with all your soul and with all your mind.' This is the first and greatest commandment. And the second is like it: 'Love your neighbor as yourself.'[b] All the Law and the Prophets hang on these two commandments."

Let's move on to how relationships affect us with regard to past personal pain and healing. We've already talked about the need to enter healthy, intimate relationships in order to achieve real healing. Intimacy doesn't mean romantic or sexual, or even with the opposite sex. Intimate in the example of God and Adam where nothing stood between them.

Even if you were a condemned inmate awaiting execution on death row in a maximum-security penal facility, you are still created with the innate desire to connect with other people and God. You might deny it, curse it or avoid it, but it's implanted in you from before your birth. Because it is a soul desire, breaking, disfiguring or denying it causes pain in life.

To promote this deep desire, God gave us a heart for love, security and significance. Before sin entered the relationship between God, Adam and Eve, He was the sole (and soul) source provider for these three needs. It was perfect, and without condition or limitation. The relationship between each was also a sacrificial, giving nature. The spiritual connection with God allowed a free flow of reassurances for these three needs.

Sin broke that communion, and thus humanity turned away from God and inward to meet his desire for love, security and significance. It also meant we stopped focusing on the sacrificial model of relationship and began the selfish desperation practice of meeting our own needs.

How about we take a moment to reflect on each of these and decide for yourself whether each and every single thread of need has been satisfied throughout your life.

It is because of our incessant need to have love, security and significance, that we are never satisfied. A better wife, more money and higher promotion are always just beyond our reach. That insatiable itch that you'll never scratch causes chaos in your spirit and an unmet longing in your soul.

Our parents also struggled with this and going back every generation until the first two folks; Adam and Eve. The separation from God because of sin cast a permanent gulf between us. It's within this dark space that your pain was created, and where you've continued to exist.

Jesus Christ came to redeem what Adam and Eve ruined. In His restoration plan, God also provided Christ as our light that not only saves but heals. Remember, Jesus didn't come to condemn but to save us. He can provide for our three deepest needs, but we must ask Him to come into our lives.

16 For God so loved the world that he gave his one and only Son, that whoever believes in him shall not perish but have eternal life. 17 For God did not send his Son into the world to condemn the world,
but to save the world through him.
John 3:16-17

Instead of spinning our wheels pursing what we've failed to achieve on our own since the beginning of time, why not put our sights on Christ? He has, does and always will meet our needs. Once we gain a level of satisfaction through the love only God provides, the security that's not based on a 401K and the significance of being a child of God, we will come to understand the source of our lifelong dissatisfaction and pain. It's within this space that true healing is discovered.

I believe in working smarter rather than harder. This is the perfect opportunity to go directly to the source of life and come to know an ultimate love, security and significance. There's no one on this earth who can provide this to us but Jesus.

Call To Action

1. Write out in detail how you would describe your life's experience with love.

2. Write out in detail how you would describe your life's experience with security.

3. Write out in detail how you would describe your life's experience with significance.

4. Write out in detail how different the world would be had Adam and Eve not fallen for temptation and sinned.

19

UNHEALTHY PERSONALITY TRAITS

"For God gave us a spirit not of fear but of power and love and self-control."
2 Timothy 1:7

I want to share a bit from my past. Our discussion about the need for love, security and significance really hit home for me. Although I knew what the topic was about and the content, just rereading and writing about it once again brought up old memories. I thought it might help you relate to our focus on relationships and this part about personality types.

I've shared my story about growing up in a dysfunctional home dominated by a silent and distant father. I also confided that we never once went to church, and although I knew there was a God, my only impression of him was what I saw in my dad. To me, God was a cold, far away intimidating force that was only there to smack me when I messed up.

Because there was no kindness, intimacy or love in my understanding of God, I did to Him what I did with my dad; I avoided them both. It left me right where you'd suspect I'd be, and it wasn't a good place for anyone. It was even worse when I tried to bring a relationship into the picture. It really wasn't fair to them once my pain overtook my desire to be a good boyfriend. Actually, they were the ones who ended up getting hurt. I'd just pack my pain and move on to the next one.

Because I had the spiritual desire for love, security and significance, I unknowingly set out to get them any way I had to. I dated, and dated, and got married and divorced, and got married on a rebound and divorced, and then over the next 20 years, I dated more, and even got engaged a few times before I ended those catastrophes-in-waiting. And finally, once I stopped relying on myself to find love, God said that He would bring me a suitable helper, but I'd have to stop and heal. He did and so did I.

My dad was a high school coach and teacher who, with my mom, raised seven kids. Times got lean, but there was always food and hand-me-down clothes. But I left home with a disquieted spirit and no sense of future direction. How could I? It was all up to me because I still hadn't come to know God. Talk about insecurity! I worked like a dog and rose up the promotional chain-of-command.

By sacrificing everything, and I mean everything for the job, I lost my wife and son to divorce. I always said work was my mistress, and the mistress stole everything from me that mattered. But what else mattered was money and saving it. Supplemental retirement, pension, 401K, CDs, everything available became my obsession so that I'd never have to worry again. Where I lacked family and spiritual security, I decided to replace it with financial security.

The stronghold of money became a boulder on my shoulders as I began to sink during a daunting financial fiasco. Almost a million dollars in debt in the blink of an eye, and no way out except to begin letting loose of the iron clad grip on my "security." My security is in and only in Jesus Christ, and not some fluctuating stock market ticker.

In sharing my testimony on significance, it's important to not confuse striving to be better with goals versus earthly consumption for the sake of easing past personal pain. At one point I grew ashamed of every degree, promotion and accomplishment I'd earned. But, after throwing my earthly crows to the ground, God showed me that what I gained on earth was to be used to serve His kingdom in heaven.

Instead of my significance being that of a child of God, I pursued academics, athletics and career advancement at a blistering pace. I recall the night I received my PhD. It's the highest academic degree available, and just over one percent of the American population has earned one.

That should've been the pinnacle of my academic achievement, right? I know you know better, because it took me from the time I received my diploma to walk down the stage, circle around the other graduates and sit down before I started hating myself again.

I remember how hard my pulse was pounding because I needed my next fix. The feeling of significance of those last 7 years in graduate school to earn a Master of Public Administration and a doctorate in cultural anthropology vanished instantly. And, just like that, I was back in darkness.

I know we all wish we'd done better or known better years earlier, but the truth is, we can't turn back the hands of time. We can either move forward toward healing from our past or remain stuck in the pit. Or maybe it's the lion's den.

One of the keys to moving forward is as we've talked about earlier. Relationships are what we were created for, and what we need to find true healing. In addition to being watchful of ourselves, we must also be aware of others with destructive personality types that will easily derail our progress. There are five basic personality types that seem to always end up in relational conflict and failure.

1. Peace at any price – these people will do anything to avoid conflict, disappointing others or having to say no. They'll also compromise who they are just to gain acceptance from someone else. Usually raised by aggressive parents who employed guilt, rejection and condemnation to gain compliance, this personality type is mistaken for agreeable

and easygoing. There is no consistency with this type because they're constantly shifting to perform. Inconsistency leads to a lack of security for their kids and spouse.
2. Jezebel – just like the woman in the Bible, these people are manipulative and controlling. They do this to have their own needs met and aren't always obvious bullies in accomplishing this. They are very covert operatives in the world of selfish manipulation.
3. Avoider – They are masters at the stiff arm. No one gets in, and everyone remains on a surface level as far as relationships go. Their fear of rejection and betrayal drives this behavior. They've been hurt in the past, and this is their defense mechanism for self-preservation. Meanwhile, they're preserving lots of pain.
4. Cold as ice – They appear to not need feelings or human contact. How they feel is not a factor in life, but what they achieve is. Workaholics are often found in this personality type. Emotional control usually lies on the surface, as they are prone to outbursts of anger.
5. Performer – They are always on a stage. Most were raised by parents who manipulated love and attention, so they learned to perform for their attention.

These personalities also cross over into multiple types employed by one person at varying degrees. Please, if you see one or a combination of these personality types in yourself, you've got to move towards recovery and restoration. These are destructive types, and not only hurt you but harm so many others.

Breaking free from your past involves recognition. Recognizing your bad personality traits is a huge part of healing. But, it's the healing process and the willingness to re-tool ourselves in God's image so that we are able to pursue sincere relationships that lead to lasting freedom.

Call To Action

1.Write out in detail how your very own testimony relates to our needs for Love, Security and Significance.

2.Write out in detail what you think your personality type is. Do you have characteristics from each or is it only one of these?

3.Write out in detail which personality traits you can and will change.

4.Write out in detail how you feel your childhood influenced your personality.

20

ANGER AND HOSTILITY

"In God, whose word I praise, in God I trust; I shall not be afraid. What can flesh do to me?"
Psalm 56:4

When I think about anger and hostility, I recall the countless times on duty when called to someone's house for disturbances. Some scenes were indescribably bloody, while others were a quiet simmer of raging calm. Both worried me, but the quiet ones flat scared me to death because they would snap eventually. And it usually ended up in someone's death.

In reality, anger doesn't always manifest itself into physical violence. We all have and experience anger differently. Anger's seldom the reason we suffer from past pain, but it's because of the past pain that we are angry.

Anger is an often-misunderstood emotion. Playing the good Christian prevents many people from expressing the truth about feeling angry. We're afraid that it's unholy to be mad. I can assure you, and I'll show you in Ephesians that it's totally cool to lose your cool. Anger is not a sin, unless you sin in your anger.

Jesus was also angry when He entered the temple and started flipping tables and chairs. The temple was His Father's house, and it was to remain holy. He even called them a den of thieves (robbers). As we say, and they probably thought back then, those were fighting words.

But, in His human emotion of anger, it produced a righteousness in a corrupt environment. This would be similar to us getting fired up and attacking someone who had attacked our family or broken into our home. But the point I want you to see is that anger is not a sin.

And Jesus entered the temple and drove out all who sold and bought in the temple, and he overturned the tables of the moneychangers and the seats of those who sold pigeons. He said to them, "It is written, 'My house shall be called a house of prayer,' but you make it a den of robbers."
Matthew 21:12-13

The problem lies more in the way we respond to, process or fail to process anger than the actual experiencing of the emotion. The apostle Paul gives us the scriptural reference that it's okay to get angry, but he also gives us the command to not sin, and a timeframe when to resolve your anger, and the consequences for failing to process and release your spirit from the anger.

"Be angry, and do not sin": do not let the sun go down on your wrath, nor give place to the devil.
Ephesians 4:26-27

I'll be the first to admit this is easier said than done. I've lain in bed many nights, angry with my wife. My heart is pumping, my body is tight, my mind keeps replaying this verse over and over until all of a sudden it stops, and my friendly neighborhood devil begins reminding me of all the things my wife has done wrong.

Whispers prompt thoughts of how much happier my life was without her. That devil even starts offering names of women better suited for me, and plants bombs of curiosity for finding them over social media. Yep, before I fall asleep hours later, I'm still just as angry, but have a plan B and C just in case I'm too angry to continue in this marriage. Yet, come morning, I can't remember why I'd gotten so mad, but those demonic bombs of impurity are beginning to implode.

Does this sound familiar? Of course, because it's Satan's number one tactic for ruining your life. Since relationships are vital to God, destroying them is vital to Satan. I also think this is why Paul was so concise in this very point. He makes it very clear what is cool, how long God will be cool with it, and what happens if it goes sideways. That's pretty easy to understand. Even for me!

We, men, have to stop shoving everything under the rug. It's creating a tipping point that either erupts little by little or all at once in an extreme violence of uncontainable destruction. Either way, you and those who care most about you wind up in the losing end. Instead try this:

1. Admit that you have anger.
2. Distinguish between healthy anger and destructive anger.
3. Allow yourself to have anger without feeling shame or guilt.
4. Understand what/who it is that causes the anger.
5. Identify who it is that you're taking your anger out on.
6. Confess your anger to God, and repent.
7. Ask forgiveness.
8. Deconstruct your source of anger to begin the process of uncovering its root cause.
9. Seek freedom from past pains, inner vows, judgments and soul ties that radiate hate.
10. Speak power over your healing by praying for God's light to eliminate the darkness that breeds anger.

Pastor Jimmy Evans talks about anchors as the most common issues we face when working to overcome anger and hostility. In order for us to overcome the destruction of anger, let's take a look at what causes most of it, and how it binds us to the sin of sinning in our anger.

Anchor 1 – Unforgiveness and Unbroken Judgments:

Seems like the topic of forgiveness pops up everywhere, and for good reason. The more we resent and judge, the angrier and more hostile we become. Remember our conversation about passing judgment over others? We often become what we resent through judging. Seek out every opportunity to forgive those who have hurt you, and those whom you have unfairly judged. This is a life changing chance.

Anchor 2 – Loss and Hurt:

The words from R.E.M.'s song, "Everybody Hurts" was on my heart as I thought over this section. Not that I'm a big fan, but the haunting chorus captured the way I'm feeling as I write this. The truth in this life is that we all experience loss and hurt.

> *Well, everybody hurts sometimes*
> *Everybody cries...*
> *So, hold on, hold on...*
> *You are not alone*

My mom passed away in 1999, and I still miss her dearly. I suffered over her loss for many years because I didn't handle the grieving process the right way. In fact, I didn't allow myself to grieve at all. And talk about a double whammy, my wife and I divorced the year before.

Anger at loss and hurt are real. People are guilty of trying to shut off the emotional framework and switching gears, but it doesn't work that way. We are human and we hurt because we also have a spiritual nature that, despite how tough of an exterior we construct, our heart is still connected to Christ.

We've got to identify situations where we've either experienced loss through death, or through divorce, distance, broken relationships or any other circumstance that separated us from our cherished ones. The feelings are there, and until we reconcile them with Christ, there is no relief. This is when healing and freedom from past and recurring pain is granted.

Anchor 3 – Fear:

The first time I read this by my pastor, Jimmy Evans, I thought it was crazy. I'm not afraid of anything. Right? I know this might sound nuts, but after I retired from law enforcement, it took just over a year for me to adjust to being a civilian. But, during that year, I developed fears about being alone, being unneeded, unwanted and basically unable to help others with their problems.

Hold on, because it sounded even crazier the first time I explained it out loud; as a result of those feelings, I developed an unhealthy fear of law enforcement, because not being one of them was what was causing the other feelings of fear. I hated driving for fear of being stopped, ticketed or arrested.

Of course, my licenses and vehicle were completely in compliance, and I have a habit of being in no rush, so speeding wasn't a possibility, but what was it? It was ultimately a fear of rejection that I had to pray through. Although I honorably retired as a Chief of Police at the date of my choice, there was still a spirit of perceived rejection from the culture of cops. God helped me to see the cause and the cure.

Anchor 4 – Ignorance:

We almost always develop a harsh reaction to what we don't understand. Sometimes it's a result of feeling intimidated by the person, item or event, while other times your anger may result in a disagreement without knowing all of the facts. It doesn't mean that we are ignorant, it means that we don't understand or have experience with whatever it is that causes us such anger and hostility.

Racism is a perfect example. Racism is a social construct, not a biological one. In other words, although anatomically similar, the coloring of a layer of skin creates a cultural divide as if we weren't even the same species.

Women are vastly more different from men than men of different races are, yet we invest the time to learn about women so that our ignorance about gender is erased. If we invested the same effort toward each race, the ignorance would be replaced by education, acceptance and appreciation. While this wasn't intended to be a discussion of race, it's the most important illustration there is for moving past the anger-producing ignorance of racism.

Anchor 5 – Spiritual Harassment:

We've already talked about the effect of demonic forces in our lives. Remember, as a Christian you cannot be possessed by the devil, but you can sure be pestered by his legion. Satan hates men because we are God's first human creation, and often the first introduction we get of what God the Father is through our dads. Simple; Satan hates you.

Causing confusion, anger and hostility stops you from creating and maintaining strong relationships. In that absence of relationships come the inability to communicate with God or others. This darkness prevents healing from our pain. When you find yourself under demonic harassment, immediately invoke God's authority over the devil and his demons.

Anchor 6 – Unrealistic and Selfish Thinking:

Do we expect more from ourselves and others than reasonable? What's reasonable you ask? Do your demands cause stress, risk or harm to others, or you? We often push ourselves beyond the safety zone for the sake of an unrealistic expectation.

The result is like overtraining in the gym: negative. Except this isn't a set of bench presses, it's life. When we seek God's will and His desires for our life, we ensure our own don't cause or continue past pain.

> *Delight yourself in the Lord,*
> *and he will give you the desires of your heart.*
> Psalm 37:4

Anchor 7 – Stress:

Stress is a silent killer. It's lethal and doesn't discriminate. Our lives are filled with it and there seems to be no escape. Unless we zero in on it and work to reduce it, the effects of anger and hostility are exponentially increased.

I used to feed off of stress. At work, the more, the better. In my personal life, my sin created much of it. Because I was surrounded by it, I thought extreme stress was the measure of a man.

The better measure is to place your priorities straight with a focus on God, spouse (if married,) kids (if you've got 'em,) and then the necessary things in life like work. God's grace provides comfort and peace that the world never can.

Cast all your anxiety on him because he cares for you.
1 Peter 5:7

Anchor 8 – Lack of Spiritual Enablement:
We as believers have been given an incredible gift of the Holy Spirit. It's as if we'd been given laptop computers back in the '80s, or before they existed. Can you imagine the power of the internet back then? I spent so much time digging through my parents' set of *Encyclopedia Britannica*. I would've loved to have just googled the information instead.

Jesus told us that the Holy Spirit would remain with us to remind us of everything Jesus has taught us. The problem is, we fail to plug in to the power of the Holy Spirit.

However, the helper, the Holy Spirit, whom the Father will send in my name, will teach you everything. He will remind you of everything that I have ever told you.
John 14:26

When we walk outside of God's grace, there is a spirit of anger and hostility because we are not practicing the fruits of the Holy Spirit: love, joy, peace, patience, kindness, goodness, faithfulness, gentleness and self-control. Instead, we're bound by the negative effects of anger over unhealed pain.

These eight anchors can be lifted and released from our lives. But it requires us to face them through prayer, forgiveness, repentance, restoration and relationships. The first relationship we must pursue is that with God our Father. Trust me, after that, everything else falls into place.

Call To Action

1. Write out in detail describing the last time you went to bed angry. Explain what caused the anger, how you felt while lying in bed, how your feelings or thoughts shifted through the night and whether you attitude changed once the anger was processed.

2. Write out in detail how you process your anger.

3. Write out a list of the eight anchors. Fill in next to each of those how they affect you, and what you will do to overcome their hold.

21

DEPRESSION

"Live as people who are free, not using your freedom as a cover-up for evil, but living as servants of God. Honor everyone. Love the brotherhood. Fear God. Honor the emperor."
1 Peter 2:16-17

Depression is another one of those tough topics to cover completely because there are so many facets of dealing with it. There are legitimate medical complications like chemical imbalances that cause depression, and there are demonic harassments as well as negative thinking.

Over 16.2 million adults in the United States, or 6.7 percent of the entire adult population have experienced depressive episodes in the course of a year. Almost half of the people diagnosed with depression are also diagnosed with an anxiety disorder. And it is estimated a full fifteen percent of all adults will experience depression at some point.

Although not all suicides are linked to depression, it is a significant partner with very close connections. In the US, suicide is the tenth leading cause of death, and the second among people ages 15-

24. This amounts to 44,000 deaths by suicide in 2016. Of those, substance abusers were six times more likely to kill themselves.

I'd be willing to bet that we all either know someone who has killed themselves or attempted to do so. It, like depression, is an epidemic in America, and the numbers continue to grow. Are you suffering from a form of depressed feelings because of the pain shackled to your back?

I want to cover a few major topics and offer solutions for allowing cracks of light to invade your darkness, until not only is your spirit filled with light, but your pain is healed as well.

Let's start with the most complex because of its medical ramifications: chemical imbalance and biogenic depression. There's no secret that we are an overly medicated society. We can thank big pharma, and doctors who don't understand pain and depression management over the excessive prescription writing that has us over-addicted and under-functioning.

Having worked undercover narcotics for 12 years, I served with the DEA Task Force, and commanded my own during that time. I have a very real insider's perspective of the damage and danger of prescription drug abuse and addiction. Depression and chronic pain were the most over-medicated claims for doctors easing their patients' claims of symptoms.

While there are legitimate causes for medication to manage chemical imbalances, one concern is that the person's significant issues of past pain are not being addressed. When there are issues of abuse, abandonment, self-hate, and the many other problems that arise from a stressed struggle through life, it's vital to combine the medical treatments with counseling (preferably Christian counseling).

Next up is something I think we all relate to, but probably never consider on an emotional level. Emotional exhaustion is no different than working hard day after day, and never giving your body the chance to rest. Eventually, your body will begin to suffer from the stress of exhaustion and performance will fade, along with an increased risk of injury.

When I first began my career in the undercover world of drugs and violent crime, I took pride in my ability to endure both physically and mentally. I used to brag that I went ten years without taking a vacation or day off. Wow was I stupid. Sure, I made lots of investigative cases, but I also suffered two divorces and lost relationships with two sons. The reality was that while almost all of those dangerous criminals are back on the streets, I'm still serving a life sentence of loss.

We need the time off to allow our emotions to relax and restore. One of the Ten Commandments we all assume is okay to break, is the one you'd think we'd clamor to observe.

> *"Remember the Sabbath day by keeping it holy.*
> *Exodus 20:8*

God is giving us a day of rest. No, it's not a day to catch up on stuff, it is a day of rest. The day is for quiet relaxation, meditation and restoration through worship. This is also the space where angers fade because of the hedge of protective silence in a Sabbath observing home.

While not the chronic medical condition, emotional exhaustion affects many if not all of us on some level. It might be the death or loss of a loved one, or a major defeat in life such as job loss or failing a test. Emotional exhaustion doesn't always follow a negative event. Emotional highs such as a wedding, childbirth or faithful experience, will have an effect of draining the tanks.

Expect this swing of emotion and combat it with time to recoup. Give yourself a break. Literally.

Unhealthy and unbiblical thinking are another cause of depressed feelings. I bet you can name someone who darkens your door by merely standing in it. Sad sacks drain us of life as quickly as they drain themselves.

I have a dear friend. He's possibly one of my best friends, but every time we talk, he brings up the same old things. It's always negative and he wants to discuss it to death. It got to a point where I explained to him that I loved him, but if we were only going to talk about the same negative things, I couldn't hang out with him anymore.

Over the following two weeks we sat in silence. It was a shame, but there was nothing to talk about unless it was that same, negative topic. While I still love him as a brother, we only call once or twice a year. I needed the break from the unhealthy conversations that created a depressed state in my emotions.

Another circumstance common among the wounded is the feeling that we're losing our mind. I've heard people share that they actually thought they were going crazy. They confessed that, although they knew better and wanted to do better, they couldn't control themselves from doing wrong.

Pornography is the most common trigger when it comes to this lack/loss of control feeling. But you have the psychological and scriptural authority to change the way your mind thinks. Yes, you can reprogram your brain. It's called neuroplasticity, and it is the process of rewiring your mind. In other words, "Thoughts that fire together; wire together."

The scriptural side of your permission to change your thinking is found in *2 Corinthians 10:4-6*. Check out the underlined for emphasis. Paul doesn't say avoid bad thoughts or try smacking them like whack-a-mole. He says take them captive.

As a career law enforcement officer, I can tell you that the act of taking someone captive is a very active and assertive process. In the same respect, you must assert the authority God has given you to capture unbiblical and unhealthy thoughts and bind them unto obedience in Christ. Not surprisingly, I found that once we started arresting bad guys at a certain place, they stopped showing up. I also discovered the same to be true when I began arresting the thoughts that caused my past personal pain to continue to thrive.

For the weapons of our warfare are not carnal but mighty in God for pulling down strongholds, casting down arguments and every high thing that exalts itself against the knowledge of God, <u>bringing every thought into captivity to the obedience of Christ</u>, and being ready to punish all disobedience when your obedience is fulfilled.
2 Corinthians 10:4-6

Let's move along to spiritual oppression. We've covered the effects of demonic harassment in detail, because it's something we don't usually sit around thinking about, and something we may not know much about. I feel like we need a reminding anchor to the reality that there is a devil on this earth, and it's not a silly horned goon dressed in red with a pitchfork.

Be alert and of sober mind. Your enemy the devil prowls around like a roaring lion looking for someone to devour.
1 Peter 5:8

And with that sobering fact, we can move forward to better understand the connection between spiritual oppression and depression. In *Isaiah 61:1-3*, depression is referred to as a heaviness, and as a spirit. The heaviness is also called "darkness." There is no coincidence that Satan's kingdom is described as one of darkness.

Isaiah doesn't just describe the heavy spirit of depression as a darkness, it also gives the cure. The garment of praise is used to describe a constant pursuit of God. Confession holds a major part in praising God. It cleans our heart, spirit and the supernatural path to an intimate relationship with our Father.

Our last major topic relative to depression and of course the pain it covers and carries is serious discouragement. I'd say what plenty of people on the fringe of clinical depressed emotions refer to as depression, is actually serious discouragement. It doesn't make it any less severe, but differences in remedies are extreme.

Most of us have experienced this. Things just not going right, and there seems like nothing we can do to stop it. That big old diesel engine of discouragement just keeps on chugging down the track. If you've been through a divorce, child custody, unemployed to name a few, it becomes very real.

God gives us the example of David, the future king of Israel, in *1 Samuel 30:6-9*. Talk about tough times, he was hunted by King Saul, exiled into tough territory, had his wife, kids and everything he owned stolen, and to top it off, his once loyal men were now talking about killing him because of the same losses they experienced.

David did what he did best. He wasted no time in turning to God, seeking God's counsel and acting upon what God instructed him to do. David encouraged himself in the Lord instead of finding a dark cave to play woe is me. Think about the last time you were seriously discouraged. How'd you bust through it?

We must make up our minds that tough times will come, and situations in life have sucked before and they are going to suck again, but the difference in then and when is the decision you make today. No matter what may come, commit that you will immediately turn to God, seek His counsel, and do what He tells you to do.

Time to act!!!

Call To Action

1. Write out in detail what you recall about the times you experienced depression.

2. Write out in detail if they were bouts of clinical depression or one of the variations described above.

3. Write out in detail how the bouts ended and whether you took affirmative action or over a period of time solved it.

4. Write out in detail struggles you face where there is a strong mental draw toward destructive behavior (porn, substances, physical abuse.)

5. Research neuroplasticity and write out in detail how you understand the process of rewiring your mind as it relates to the list from #4.

22

ADDICTION

"For we do not want you to be ignorant, brothers, of the affliction we experienced in Asia. For we were so utterly burdened beyond our strength that we despaired of life itself. Indeed, we felt that we had received the sentence of death. But that was to make us rely not on ourselves but on God who raises the dead. He delivered us from such a deadly peril, and He will deliver us. On Him we have set our hope that he will deliver us again."
2 Corinthians 1:8-10

Addiction is similar to the term, depression. No one wants to deal with it, or even admit that it has a hold in our life. Admitting it, much less talking to others about it surely has to make us look weak among our lion herd. Right?

Well, I'm not going to tell you what you already know. It makes people uncomfortable when bringing it up. That's why it's such an awesome weapon in Satan's arsenal. I worked undercover narcotics operations for twelve years, and the work addiction was not looked upon with compassion. When it came time for me to face the reality of my own addictions, it was a challenge.

Merriam-Webster defines addiction as the quality or state of being addicted. How much do you love that definition (yes, sarcasm)? Another is the compulsive need for and use of a habit-forming substance (such as heroin, nicotine, or alcohol.) Persistent, compulsive use of a substance known by the user to be harmful.

I've never met anyone who chose to be an addict. Whether it was drugs, food, sex, alcohol, relationships or eating paper, no one ever wanted their life controlled by a substance or action.

Not only do addicts require ministry, but those who are an important part of their lives also require care. We'll talk about codependents later, but for now, please accept that addictive behavior affects everyone within your circle. We might think we've fooled them, but trust me, they are aware, they are suffering, and they are wanting you to get help.

Most addictive behavioral patterns find their roots in dysfunctional family homes. These homes are unhealthy and fail to meet our three most basic needs. Since we've discussed them in detail earlier, I'll skim over for the reminder.

We were created with a desire for love, security and significance. God designed our relationship with Him so that He'd meet each of the three needs. He is love; therefore, the relationship is one of ultimate love. Security is found in God's presence, as he is a protective and providing Father. The significance of being a child of God the Father is as important as one could ever achieve.

As we've discussed, Adam's break from God's close communion in the Garden of Eden separated us from all three of those needs. Instead of living an outward serving and loving life, we've been forced to find all three of these elsewhere.

Dysfunctional homes fail to provide for love, security and significance. Because the desire is spirit-led, we cannot choose to not want them met, so we seek to satisfy them by looking outside the home. The absence of these needs also causes pain that continues to burrow and grow until we're forced to medicate it.

We've also talked about deadening our pain with the same acts, substances and behaviors that quickly lead to an all-consuming addiction. It's a sly, but harsh transition. We don't realize we're suffering at home until our need for love, security and significance begins to take hold of our soul. Maybe we act out, or turn inward because the lack of family love, leadership and acceptance hurts until it harms.

By the time we're old enough to understand that we're not satisfied, happy or even content, we seek out ways to minimize the pain of not experiencing the love, security or significance from our family. This is where we enter the addiction funnel. I'll go over each phase that leads to addiction, so you may spot a place where you are, or where you've been. Prayerfully, if you see something familiar, you stop the train before it barrels forward.

Stage 1 – Experimentation:

Although addiction is complex, the beginning usually starts with curiosity and peer pressure. Whether it's pornography, alcohol or heroin, no one sees the perceived danger of the behavior at this early point. It might not even be associated with the need to numb your personal pain, but because it alters your state of being, the allure of escape begins.

Stage 2 – Unconscious Acceptance:

You have accepted that the use of your substance, behavior or actions are now a normal, and beneficial part of your life. You've embraced the stimuli as you own but claim you can walk away at any time. By this stage, you've connected the dots that your pain doesn't affect you while engaged with your acting out. You are empowered by the ability to control your escape mechanism.

Stage 3 – Usage Increase:

This is the point of no turning back. Your obsession has quietly taken control of you, while you indeed thought you were still in control of it. You no longer see it as something you master, but something that masters you. There's no living without it, and you begin adjusting your life to accommodate your addiction.

Stage 4 – Deepest Addiction:

Your life comes second to the obsession. Actually, your life is only lived to feed the obsession. No one matters above the stimuli and you'll stop at nothing to bump up the fading euphoria that is never as wonderful as the first time you engaged in it. You will do anything to get your next fix and will hurt anyone standing in your way.

Let's revisit something we've discussed earlier on the topic of healing. It comes in one of two ways. Yes, God can miraculously heal you in an instant, and the desire, compulsion or obsession will never tempt you again. Or, healing can be a process as in a work in progress.

In the process that is drawn out over time, there are resources that are available and valuable. Medical treatment facilities are important if required. For example, in a case of heroin addiction, before methadone can be prescribed, a medical doctor is required.

During the process of recovering from a physical addiction, support groups and prayers from loved ones are vital to breaking free from the chains of addiction. In the process of healing, there are four areas of required change:

1. Physical Addiction – The source of obsession doesn't matter, although some actions are much more dangerous to your health than others. If your addiction is physical, the goal is to address that before any other issues such as unhealthy relationships, emotions, or thought life can be repaired. Substance use must be stopped before moving forward in the healing process.
2. Healing of Emotions – Repairing emotions is tough. Avoiding pain is what set us on an unhealthy path to begin with. The emotional damage caused because of the past pain must be addressed. Rejection is a main source of the hurt. Working to identify where your pain began, is a great place to start with forgiveness so you may experience freedom from the emotion and the pain.
3. Lifestyle – Your life reflects your addiction. Your friends, activities and job, if you manage to hold on to one, all change to ensure your addiction is top priority. In order to

heal, everything must change. Yes, especially your circle of influencers. I love this saying, "Show me your friends, and I'll show you your future."

4. Life Skills – Addicts become very savvy at adapting so as to feed their next fix. There is a desperation in their edge that makes them take risks and fight to survive for the sake of satisfying their addiction. Once they are free of their addiction, most find themselves unable to function in the ordinary life activities. For however many years there has been an addict's fog, that many years no maturation evolved in your life. It makes addicts uneasy and wanting to return to what they see as the simple life.

The key is to identify whether or not we have developed an addiction. Addictions rarely just happen. During my time spent assigned to a drug task force, I have met people who were curious to try a drug, and after one time, they were hooked, but the high majority of occasions, addictions began as described above. Most of those times we didn't even know one was forming until a tipping point that forced us to face it head on.

The beauty is that through Jesus Christ we can know freedom from painful pasts and all of the ill-gotten behaviors caused by it.

Therefore, if anyone is in Christ, the new creation has come:
The old has gone, the new is here!
2 Corinthians 5:17

Call To Action

1. Write out in detail what addictive or compulsive behaviors you are dealing with.

2. Write out in detail your earliest memories of accessing your addictive substance, product, behavior, etc.

3. Write out in detail what effects addiction has had on your personal and professional life.

4. Write out in detail what steps you have taken to break free from addiction.

23

ARMORED FOR SPIRITUAL WARFARE

"Since therefore the children share in flesh and blood, He Himself likewise partook of the same things, that through death He might destroy the one who has the power of death, that is, the devil, and deliver all those who through fear of death were subject to lifelong slavery."
Hebrews 2:14-15

I love the Bible's imagery of war, battle, and armoring up for the fight. God calls it like it is; it's a war, and as the saying goes, war is hell. Well, in this case, we are at war with hell's legion of demons. But, unlike earthly encounters where victory is never certain until the battle is done, we already know who raised the flag of victory.

Jesus Christ reigns supreme because He's already won the war. And by His authority over Satan, we are victors too. Then why are we still struggling you might ask, and sometimes it feels like we're losing? It's simple, the devil doesn't throw victory parties for believers. He's also tenacious and refuses to give up until he's finally locked away in the lake of fire.

> *And the devil who had deceived them was cast into the lake of fire and brimstone, where the beast and the false prophet are; and they shall be tormented day and night for ever and ever.*
> Revelation 20:10

So, until then, we have to care for the fortresses we've constructed for God's kingdom and our freedom. The fortress of spiritual warfare is something many figure they'll just avoid for the time being. The reality of a spirit realm still seems a little too made-for-movies. But the reality is, we live in both a natural and supernatural realm. Our daily existence is in the natural, and this is where every ounce of our past pain originated. When we pray and communicate with the Holy Spirit, we enter the spiritual realm.

God gives us everything we need for spiritual warfare. It's His suit of armor, and it is invincible. When I first was appointed as my city's chief of police, one if the chaplains would regularly visit with me. He'd explain that my job wasn't to fight crime, but it was a supernatural battle against demonic forces in the city. I believed him when he said it, but I really began to believe him when I began to live it.

Our battle to gain independence from our past isn't against other people. No one can make you live in your memories. Sure, they can remind you of certain times in your life, but they don't hold the power to return you. These shackles remain entrenched in your mind and is why transforming your thought-life is critical to freedom.

If you are battling people over your access to your past pain, it might be an indicator that you have not yet forgiven them. If that's the case, you've got to stop here, and forgive anyone who holds the keys to your healing.

So, let's charge forward and deconstruct God's armor to understand exactly what it is. I've underlined points of emphasis so we can discuss.

> 10 Finally, my brethren, be strong in the Lord and in the power of His might. 11 Put on the <u>whole armor of God</u>, that ye may be able to <u>stand against</u> the wiles of the devil. 12 For we wrestle <u>not against flesh and blood</u>,

but against principalities, against powers, against the <u>rulers of the darkness of this world</u>, against spiritual wickedness in high places.
13 Therefore, take unto you the whole armor of God, that ye may be able to withstand in the evil day and, having done all, to stand. 14 Stand therefore, having your <u>loins girded about with truth</u>, and having on the <u>breastplate of righteousness</u>, 15 and <u>your feet shod with the preparation</u> of the Gospel of peace.
16 Above all, take the <u>shield of faith</u>, wherewith ye shall be able to quench all the fiery darts of the wicked. 17 And take the <u>helmet of salvation</u> and the <u>sword of the Spirit</u>, which is the Word of God,
18 praying always with all prayer and supplication in the Spirit, and watching thereunto with all perseverance and supplication for all saints.
Ephesians 6:10-18

Important points:

1. Our fight is with the devil.
2. Devil's weapon is deception. Girding your loins (belt) of truth defeats lies and suspicious.
3. Breastplate of Righteousness defends our most vital organs, and defeats Satan's deadly tactic of casting shame and condemnation.
4. Our feet shod are the spikes roman soldiers wore to improve their stable footing in battle. Shod in peace is to have harmony with God.
5. Shield of Faith protects us from the fiery darts launched by the devil. His darts are pain, shame and defeat.
6. Helmet of Salvation protects your other vital organ; your brain. Thought life is where Satan finds the cracks to tempt you or deceive you through division. The helmet guards your thought-life.
7. Sword of the Spirit is God's Word. This is your offensive weapon so that once the devil comes at you, like he did Jesus in the wilderness, you will repel him with God's truths.

Prayer is an important fortress, and it is also the direct line of communications with our 4-star general in the times of warfare. God is your hope and your salvation. Remaining in close contact with Him during the battle will ensure your victory over the enemy.

Praise and worship are another tool in your arsenal for repelling the devil's advances. Satan hates worship and praise. I mean he hates it. The disciples Paul and Silas were locked up with no hope for release. Acts 16:25 tells of the ground erupting and the prison doors shaken open while they sang out praise from the deepest pit of the prison.

King David, who had faced so many dilemmas also praised and worshipped God with every fiber of his being. He was delivered from the hands of death on several occasions during his times of offering praise in his pain.

4 Look and see, there is no one at my right hand; no one is concerned for me.
I have no refuge; no one cares for my life.
5 I cry to you, Lord; I say, "You are my refuge, my portion in the land of the living."
6 Listen to my cry, for I am in desperate need; rescue me from those who pursue me, for they are too strong for me.
7 Set me free from my prison, that I may praise your name.
Then the righteous will gather about me because of your goodness to me.
Psalm 142:4-7

The last weapon for your spiritual fortress is to persevere. Victory in battle is seldom swift, and while the initial blows may seem to dictate a conqueror, perseverance is the key. Do you know how long the Hundred Year War lasted? Actually, it's not a trick question, but it lasted one hundred and sixteen years. War is not only hell, but it can be long lasting.

We can look at Job for an example of persevering through pain. He'd lost everything except his faith in God. Like us, it may seem the hurting will never stop, but God has never once forsaken us or forgotten us. As we've been talking about, our healing is a process, and like Job, there is an end in the fighting and a blessing awaits.

Our past pain has been attached to us because we've not yet worked through the process. There is nothing that God cannot heal. And by heal, I mean, either miraculous intervention, or over a period of time as you draw closer to Him.

God touched my heart years ago when I saw the story of Eva Moses Kor, a Holocaust survivor. She and her twin sister were subjected to horrific human experimentation under the direction of Josef Mengele at the Auschwitz concentration camp. Although she lost both parents and two older sisters, she and her twin miraculously survived the torture and medical experiments. In 2015, she travelled back to Germany to testify at the trial of one of the doctors responsible for her and her sister's horror. She personally forgave him, and the Nazis for what was done to her.

This is perseverance!

If we armor up, pray, praise and persevere, we will be delivered from the attacks that have stopped us from seeking healing for our past pain.

Submit yourselves, then, to God. Resist the devil, and he will flee from you.
James 4:7

Call To Action

1. Write out in detail what your spiritual armor looks like in a natural sense.

2. Write out a situation where you thought hope was lost, but you continued to praise God for every little step until you'd come through it.

3. Write out in detail an experience where God's healing or grace took longer than you had hoped, but when you had been delivered, what lesson was learned.

24

YOUR DAILY WALK

"Because he holds fast to Me in love, I will deliver him; I will protect him, because he knows My name. When he calls to Me, I will answer him; I will be with him in trouble; I will rescue him and honor him."
Psalm 91:14-15

We've carried around backpacks full of past personal pain for so long we've become hardened against most emotions, hope and help. Like me, I just assumed I was broken, and tried to figure out the best way to get along without hurting too many other people. I wasn't very good at either.

When I broke free from my past of personal pain, it was like a flood of emotional reality. I'd discolored my past through a lens of fake memories, and false justifications for the very people responsible for preventing that harm. Forgiveness didn't come easy, but when it did, I was truly free from my past.

But like any victory in battle, you don't just stick a flag in the ground and celebrate. We must defend our progress and protect ourselves from new attacks. Trust me, if the devil is on your tail, it isn't to wish you well. It shows that you've moved away from his clutches and closer to God. Otherwise, he'd leave you alone as you wallow in his miserable control.

Fortress building is how earthly kingdoms survived conquering new ground and maintaining their presence, and it's how you'll defend your newfound territory where the pain of your past stays there; in the past.

The first fortress for you to construct is a daily walk with Jesus Christ. If there is to be true freedom from your past, then your personal relationship is the singularly most important aspect of your efforts. Without Christ, there is no lasting freedom from pain, nor is there genuine healing.

God's salvation is a gift. There's nothing in this life that can earn it or deserve it. Trying to do so is an insult to the gift-giver: God. How we protect that gift also says volumes about how we feel for the gift giver. So, these fortresses not only protect our freedom, but they show God the Father that we do love Him for the gift of salvation through His son Jesus Christ.

For it is by grace you have been saved, through faith—and this is not from yourselves, it is the gift of God—not by works, so that no one can boast.
Ephesians 2:8-9

Any good relationship requires work. It's not uncommon for us, men, to come into a relationship with Christ as our Lord and Savior, only to have the initial excitement and fire for Him to fade until we're back at a point before we knew Him. Why? Unless we're mentored on the three most basic ways of pursuing that relationship, it'll diminish in intensity.

Praying, Reading, and Submitting are the keys to a vibrant Christ-led life of freedom.

It's easy to get overwhelmed and intimidated by the unconceivable sovereignty of God. It blows my mind that He created it all, yet He still wants to know me. I mean really, who am I that He would want to pursue a relationship? I always think back to King David, who asked the very same questions.

> *Then King David went in and sat before the Lord, and he said:*
> *"Who am I, Sovereign Lord, and what is my family,*
> *that you have brought me this far?*
> *2 Samuel 7:18*

The truth is, relationship is the very reason God created us. So, yes, God does want to be our best bud, and if we'd stop running, ducking and trying to jive Him, we'd enjoy a relationship that held more promise and blessings than ever imaginable. That closeness comes through communication: prayer.

God not only wants us to pray, but He promises to hear and answer our prayers if we come by faith. For people like us who have struggled and come into the light of Christ for healing freedom, we might wonder why, if we ask God to set us back on track, doesn't He answer our prayers.

God does hear your prayer, and like we've talked about before, there are two ways of healing: instant miracle and by process. For those of us who went through an entire process, it doesn't mean God gave more weight to others' prayer, or mine weren't strong enough.

It meant for me that there was so much past to get past, that I would've missed processing and sorting out relationships, feelings and a clear perspective going forward. God guards our hearts, and I know without a doubt that had everything been dumped on me at once, I would've been devastated instead of liberated.

The next step to reinforcing an invincible fortress is to read God's word every day. The Bible is unlike any book. You don't read the Bible; the Bible reads you. It makes God's word come alive, and plants His very specific desires for your live, deep into your heart.

What you water your soul with will bear the fruit of that word. Years ago, I used to read the news the instant I woke up. Of course, everything is so biased and negative, that even before I'd stepped foot out of bed, my attitude would reflect a hardened, pessimistic tone.

Reading God's word in the morning's quiet time sets my head and heart apart if for only a moment in time, but it positions my attitude for the remainder of the day.

The third, and final part of structuring your fortress is yielding to the Holy Spirit. Unfortunately, the Holy Spirit is like the George Harrison of the Beatles. Unknown and often forgotten for the sake of God the Father and Jesus Christ, the Holy Spirit is the third and equally part of the holy trinity.

The Holy Spirit's role is usually misunderstood, and therefore not given the attention of pursuing a relationship with Him. In John 16:7-15, Jesus tells His disciples that He must go so that the Comforter may come. He explains who and what the Holy Spirit is, and why it's necessary. Today, the Holy Spirit's role is just as vital and alive as when He fell upon the people at Pentecost.

If you haven't up to this point, please begin to pursue a relationship with the Holy Spirit. You aren't cutting God out of your worship by doing so, you are plugging directly into His power. The Holy Spirit gives us God's power (Acts 1:8) and fills us with the character of Christ (Galatians 5:22) so we may have gifts for ministry (1 Corinthians 12) to comfort us (John 16:7).

I want to share 1 Corinthians 12 with you because it's the complete explanation of who the Holy Spirit is. This is so important to understand because I've known people who thought the Holy Spirit was an angel or a myth. Trust me, but more important, accept God's word, that the power of God resides in the presence of the Holy Spirit. I've underlined the gifts of and through the Holy Spirit for reference.

1 Now in regard to spiritual gifts, brothers, I do not want you to be unaware. 2 You know how, when you were pagans, you were constantly attracted and led away to mute idols. 3 Therefore, I tell you that nobody speaking by the spirit of God says, "Jesus be accursed." And no one can say, "Jesus is Lord," except by the holy Spirit.
4 There are different kinds of spiritual gifts but the same Spirit; 5 there are different forms of service but the same Lord; 6 there are different workings

> *but the same God who produces all of them in everyone. 7 To each individual the manifestation of the Spirit is given for some benefit.*
> *8 To one is given through the Spirit the expression of <u>wisdom</u>; to another the expression of <u>knowledge</u> according to the same Spirit;*
> *9 to another <u>faith</u> by the same Spirit; to another gifts of <u>healing</u> by the one Spirit;*
> *10 to another <u>mighty deeds</u>; to another <u>prophecy</u>; to another <u>discernment of spirits</u>; to another varieties of <u>tongues</u>; to another <u>interpretation of tongues</u>.*
> *11 But one and the same Spirit produces all of these, distributing them individually to each person as he wishes.*
> *12 As a body is one though it has many parts, and all the parts of the body, though many, are one body, so also Christ. 13 For in one Spirit we were all baptized into one body, whether Jews or Greeks, slaves or free persons, and we were all given to drink of one Spirit.*
> 1 Corinthians 12:1-13

These are the three most important things you can do to ensure that you do break free from your past, and that you will stay free. These building blocks will make your fortress invincible against the attacks of the enemy. Please commit to the time to pray, read and submit daily. You will come to know the Holy Spirit as your best ally and friend.

Call To Action

1. Write out in detail what you understand praying to be. Think through this and try to deconstruct how you think about prayer in your life.

2. Write out in detail what you like and don't like about reading the Bible. What draws you to it or keeps you away from it.

3. Write out in detail what role you understand the Holy Spirit to play in the Holy Trinity.

4. Write out in detail how and when you will make the time to pray, read and submit on a daily basis.

25

A TRANSFORMED MIND

"He has now reconciled in His body of flesh by His death, in order to present you holy and blameless and above reproach before Him."
Colossians 1:22

I've been fortunate to have traveled outside of the United States, and to experienced ancient ruins and early century forts, castles and blockades built as defensive weapons against attacks of war. Some of the most incredible structures imaginable were never once tested in combat, and still sit peacefully at attention over a time gone by.

Why weren't they used? Because their very presence, through preparation, served as a greater deterrent than any number of warriors or weapons. They were steady in getting ready and the enemy knew they weren't up against some village of rock throwers. It's no wonder most of these kingdoms and countries survive still today.

When we talk about readying our fortress with praying, reading the Bible and submitting to the Holy Spirit, we are building a defensive posture in our daily walk with Christ. The further we pull away from the bowels of Satan's suppression of past personal pain, the more involved he and his demons become in getting your back into a crooked environment.

Also, not to say that every bad day, flat tire or headache is of the devil, but strengthening your tower will also help defend you from getting distracted by life's everyday drama. Now, I can't promise you won't get upset by your favorite sports team's loss, but your fortress is your protection.

I've purposefully mentioned defensive protection because I want to now talk about offensive weapons. The most important weapon you have in the fight for your freedom is your mind. It is an incredible machine and a supercomputer that by all scientific estimates is only performing at ten percent of its intended capacity. As magnificent as the human brain is, it served as a blessing and a curse to most of us.

Our ability to transform our mind is the next important piece of the fortress-building process. The fuel for the shift from a carnal-driven organism into a spiritual weapon is God's word. There are a few sayings that apply here; Garbage in, garbage out is one of them that holds true.

Feeding our brain with the liberal media's diet of movies, television, news and social media causes the brain to operate in a chaotic stream of sex, violence and an abnormal appreciation of the world we live in and others imagined. Cursing, and talking about the vile things of this world burns brain potential, as does gossip and speaking wicked of others.

Love not the world, neither the things that are in the world. If any man love the world, the love of the Father is not in him.
1 John 2:15

We've touched on this earlier in the book, but neuroplasticity is so important that you understand and trust it's real and possible for you to transform your mind from a spiritual platform.

The brain's own process of rewiring, or reprogramming itself is the real deal, so dig deeper it out if you want more information. But, the reality of it is, you have the power to retrain your brain. Let's back up to the earlier saying about firing and wiring (*Thoughts that fire together, wire together.*) People struggling with pornography tell me they have tried to stop their consumption, but their cravings are too strong. They're trapped in a rut, with no hope of freedom from an addiction caused by early pain.

A porn addict's brain actually experiences change thanks to chemical activity released while craving and then actually watching pornography. Thanks to the chemical reactions, your brain rewires itself to focus on satisfying its need for visual stimulation. Soon, it only desires the fantasy stimulation, and real, physical sex has little to no appeal.

I've been told that they were addicted to porn because that's the way God made them. Can I tell you that's a load of junk? You were not born with an innate need for porn. Porn didn't become an issue until exposure, and with that exposure soon came the addiction. Why? Because that was what you fed your brain, so it programmed itself with the fuel it was being fed.

The great news is, the brain can be rewired. It depends on what fuel you use to super charge it. Prayer to get your brain into a supernatural nature is the primer, and daily Bible readings are the high-octane fuel that gets your thought-life steered in the right direction by the Holy Spirit.

Transforming our mind serves the purpose for connecting us into Christ today and in the future as we grow closer in our walk with Him. Our thoughts are also the tether to our past, and tap into the painful memories we recall, or unconsciously suppress. Thoughts are our gateway to the past.

We cannot truly be free and connected to Christ if we continue fueling our thought-life with things of this world. Satan will continue to flood our minds with distractions about failures, doubts, past sins although God has long forgiven and forgotten them, and new temptations to lure our thoughts away from the word and the works of God.

Let's consider the devil's favorite attack tactic; messing with our mind. He got into Eve's head smack dab in the middle of paradise. In

Luke 4:1-13, he also tempted Jesus in the wilderness for forty days. Satan couldn't and wouldn't lay a finger on Him, but he gave it his all to tempt Jesus into thinking about sinning. Of course, Christ was never tempted or considered falling for the lies, but what's important for us to know is the experience was also a mind game.

The devil promises stuff he doesn't own and can't deliver. Why do we call him the father of lies, yet accept what he says as the gospel truth? When he plants doubt over our recovery and freedom from the past, we succumb to his lies. When we commit to seeking help for what hurts us, he tells us that it's a secret, so we keep our mouths shut and suffer in silence.

There's no need to sit on the sidelines where your thought-life is concerned. Paul makes it very clear that we are to take an active, possessive posture over anything entering our minds. Don't just allow it to noodle around in there or wait for it to take hold before trying to redirect your thoughts. Snatch the illegitimate thought up and own it by bringing it into submission to Christ.

We demolish arguments and every pretension that sets itself up against the knowledge of God, and we take captive every thought to make it obedient to Christ.
2 Corinthians 10:5

There are so many benefits to transforming your mind into a spiritual fortress for your war against a painful past. Consider what we've discussed, and I pray you will gain an appreciation for the role of your mind in the war for independence from past pain.

Think about it!

Call To Action

1. Write out in detail what thoughts slip into your mind the most that you'd have trouble explaining to your wife, loved ones and Jesus.

2. Write out in detail how you handle those thoughts.

3. Write out in detail what fuel you use to feed your thought life.

4. Write out in detail what information you can meditate to recharge spiritual thinking.

26

ACCOUNTABILITY

"Out of my distress I called on the Lord; the Lord answered me and set me free."
Psalm 118:5

I was sitting in the back seat of a friend's pickup truck as we returned to the church's parking lot after lunch. The friend in the passenger seat hoped out so we could pull in closer to a barrier which gave us room to get out on the driver's side. It was just us two left in the truck. He looked back at me through his rear-view mirror and asked a question that took me by surprise.

"Do you mentor men?"

"No."

We both got out of his truck in silence. I regretted my response, but at the time I had not ever mentored anyone. I thought to myself, who am I to hold anyone else accountable? I'd had my own problems and felt lucky enough to escape without having them destroy me.

Soon I learned that it wasn't my job to hold others accountable, as much as it is for me to help hold themselves accountable. Too much of the other way, and it devolves into judgment of someone else's behavior. Being an accountability partner wasn't what had scared me, it was not understanding the difference in the relationship between two people. Accountability is an honest reckoning of self-judgment, while a partner is there to monitor with an objective perspective, and gentle, encouraging words.

So, what is accountability? A few people I know through the ministry used to describe it as ratting yourself out to God. I used to laugh and tell them that would be confession, but they were close. Although I knew the term ratting out was more of a joke amongst them, the intention of making known what was done, was absolutely on point.

So, then each of us will give an account of himself to God.
Romans 14:12

In the context of breaking free from our past of personal pain, the term accountability conjures up what my friends used to joke about. The negative connotation associated comes from disciplinary uses. Back in grade school, on the job, civil and criminal codes, and in church, all we've ever known is the reactive nature of being held accountable.

No wonder no one wants to hold themselves accountable. I guess my friends were right on another level. When applied in a negative "gotcha" after the fact, it loses its appeal, and application for the sake of what we're working to accomplish.

Let's look at accountability another way.

What if we instead looked at accountability in a positive light? If instead of it being a tool to retro-discover failures, we front-load success by clearly identifying the expectations ahead of time, and then applying accountability measures as a means to progressively monitor and mentor the entirety of the journey.

I was not, and never will be a good runner. Especially not a fast runner. Even while training for triathlons and half marathons, my running philosophy was start slow, end slower. But in running, the timed splits are vital. They are a front-end goal for potential success.

Let's say you are running the mile on a standard high school track. That will be four laps until you collapse into a heap of air-sucking gratitude that it's done. But if you want to set a new record, then you know there is a goal pace for running each of the four laps.

Running slow around lap two doesn't mean failure, it just means you have two more laps to pick up the pace so that by the checkered flag, you'll have brought yourself back into alignment aimed at victory.

Do they actually wave a checkered flag in running? I'm not sure, but I hope you get the idea. Accountability is important, and scripturally necessary for keeping ourselves on the path toward obtaining whatever goal we've set before us.

We also achieve our goals more often when we work with an accountability partner. Not a task master, or judge, or disciplinarian, but in the biblical description of a person who cares about you and is as invested in your success as you are.

Brothers, if anyone is caught in any transgression, you who are spiritual should restore him in a spirit of gentleness. Keep watch on yourself, lest you too be tempted. Bear one another's burdens, and so fulfill the law of Christ.
For if anyone thinks he is something, when he is nothing, he deceives himself. But let each one test his own work, and then his reason to boast will be in himself alone and not in his neighbor. For each will have to bear his own load.
Galatians 6:1-5

I know you might prefer holding yourself accountable as opposed to opening yourself up to others. It's embarrassing to ask for help with a personal problem. It can be downright mortifying to share the details, but God encourages us to not only hold each other accountable, but to also confess our sins to one another for healing.

> Therefore, confess your sins to one another and pray for one another, that you may be healed. The prayer of a righteous person has great power as it is working.
> *James 5:16*

Don't allow the shame whispered into your ear by Satan to continue your failed attempts to break free. Hiding your sin, addiction and pain from others is exactly what the enemy wants you to do. Suffering in silence is not living. Although not scripture, I use this quote often as it once helped me to realize that I didn't have the resources to do it myself.

"We can't solve problems by using the same kind of thinking we used when we created them."

~ Albert Einstein

We need each other. One-on-one, prayer groups, small groups, online, or the many other opportunities to submit your goals of breaking free from your past pains before other believers, is a great way of increasing your ability to stop the destructive behaviors that have shackled you to the past, while encouraging the positive changes that ensure freedom.

Please, get connected.

Call To Action

1. Write out in detail what your experiences with accountability have been; good or bad.

2. Write out in detail what goals you would share with an accountability partner.

3. Write out in detail what goals you would not share with an accountability partner.

4. Write out in detail why you would not share anything you didn't match on the list above.

5. Write out in detail a list of men, and their contact information, that you would feel close enough to for serving as an accountability partner.

27

BOUNDARIES

Grace and peace be multiplied to you in the knowledge of God and of Jesus our Lord; seeing that His divine power has granted to us everything pertaining to life and godliness, through the true knowledge of Him who called us by His own glory and excellence. For by these He has granted to us His precious and magnificent promises, so that by them you may become partakers of the divine nature, having escaped the corruption that is in the world by lust.
2 Peter 1:2-4

"It was just one peek," said one of the men I worked with.

"And what happened?" I asked.

"I relapsed." Todd (not his real name) sighed.

There was no judgment or condemnation of this man. Todd had struggled with pornography since he was twelve. He was rejected by his mother when he sought her rescue after repeated sexual assaults by his stepfather. Abandoned emotionally, Todd was left empty, aching and alone. After Todd and his mother were dumped by the sex offender, the only ones who made him feel loved and safe were the actors in his pornography.

Todd had worked with counselors for years to overcome his addiction. He'd broken free for about two years and had managed to forgive his mother and stepfather for the horror inflicted on a once young and promising future. Todd connected with me about six months before his relapse because he'd begun to feel alone following his second divorce and sought an accountability partner to help him stay on the rails.

One of the first things I helped Todd establish were boundaries. He was already familiar with the concept, so it wasn't as much of a challenge to get him to identify them, as it was to encourage him not to cross over them. That conversation I began this section with was the last conversation Todd and I would have.

Boundary setting can be seen as an insult and restriction to their manliness. We are independent after all. Like a yard dog with an electronic fence, we don't like being boxed in. Of course, this is also what gets us into most of our troubles. My wife had a great way of explaining that you create boundaries to protect what you love, while keeping the threats on the outside.

She is correct. Boundaries are meant for our protection. Cells are created for our confinement. There was only one boundary at the very beginning of creation. Adam and Eve were free to roam the entirety of paradise. Talk about a sweet deal, they were placed over everything God had personally created.

> And God blessed them, and God said unto them, Be fruitful, and multiply, and replenish the earth, and subdue it: and have dominion over the fish of the sea, and over the fowl of the air, and over every living thing that moveth upon the earth.
> *Genesis 1:28*

Except for the one and only boundary, Adam and Eve had nothing to worry about. God made it easy and told Adam to eat from any tree in the garden. And in paradise, there had to be some incredibly delicious fruit trees. But, back to that single exception of the tree of knowledge of good and evil. With that one boundary set for everyone's own good, God left them to enjoy the literal fruits of His labor.

15 The Lord God took the man and put him in the garden of Eden to work it and keep it. 16 And the Lord God commanded the man, saying, "You may surely eat of every tree of the garden, 17 but of the tree of the knowledge of good and evil you shall not eat, for in the day that you eat of it you shall surely die."
Genesis 2:15-17

You see, just like Todd, their attention didn't seek the freedom of choice and the unlimited number of other alternatives. No, Satan wants you to cross that line. He can't shove you across it, but he sure will get inside your head to consume your thoughts with nothing else but what's been set outside of your boundary.

Todd was no different than Adam, and they're no different than any of us. We want what we can't have. But there are reasons why we can't have certain "fruits," and of course, there are consequences when we take that bite out of those that are forbidden.

Following up on the example of Adam and Eve, not only did they violate the boundary and lose their intimate connection with God, but there was another boundary established that they were forbidden to cross. Of course, it was the entrance to the Garden of Eden, and this time God ensured it with the help of an angel and flaming sword. Yes, some consequences are greater than others.

After he drove the man out, he placed on the east side of the Garden of Eden cherubim and a flaming sword flashing back and forth to guard the way to the tree of life.
Genesis 3:24

How fired up do you think Satan was once he saw Adam and Eve on the outside of paradise and God's will? Yep, the same amount of happiness that he felt when Todd logged in to that porn site.

We've got to either set boundaries for ourselves, have help in setting them, or have someone set them for us. There are different scenarios, but all include respecting the purpose of boundaries, and the potential consequences for breaching them.

When we look at the big picture, I'm not sure why we, men, are so averse to the idea of boundaries. They are everywhere from speed limits on the highway to number of calories on a diet. Boundaries shouldn't be seen as limits to our fun, but standard bearers for achieving success.

Where are you in need of boundaries?
- Pornography
- Alcohol
- Drugs
- Foods
- Sex
- Texting or social media
- Locations such as strip clubs or bars

I was talking with a counselor one day and he shared a story about a client who had overcome his bondage to sexual sin. The man had spent his life savings at strip clubs and on prostitutes. The counselor said the man was so excited that he'd been free for a while and wanted to pay it forward. The man's idea was to preach the gospel to the strippers and hookers at the clubs in his area.

The counselor laughed and said that was a resounding no. He had to explain to the man that he'd forfeited the ability to witness to women in those environments, because they were beyond his boundary. In the world of recovery and freedom, you really can't have your cake and eat it too.

I suggest you get help in establishing boundaries to ensure you break free and stay free from the pain of your past. It's easy to focus on avoiding the obvious, but there are many other areas you may not realize that remain threats to your freedom.

Without an objective perspective, you may not see the people closest to you that serve as triggers for breaking boundaries, locations that remind you of the "good old days," or activities that are just waiting to reel you back in. Although we've already talked about the difficulty in confiding in others, it's going to be necessary for identifying a set of boundaries that are for your good and your success.

Here's to protecting the good stuff.

Call To Action

1. Write out in detail all boundaries you already have in place.

2. Write out in detail whether you've honored or broken each boundary, and if broken, include a detailed explanation of why.

3. Write out in detail what boundaries you need to set in place, and why.

4. Write out the names and contact information of the people in your life that would be best for helping you establish boundaries.

28

CONSEQUENCES

For God so loved the world, that He gave his only Son, that whoever believes in Him should not perish but have eternal life. For God did not send His Son into the world to condemn the world, but in order that the world might be saved through Him.
John 3:16-17

I always told my kids, "Decisions and Consequences."

As they grew older, they'd laugh and say, we know, decisions and consequences. Those two words brought almost as much joy as my three favorite words, "I love you."

Those two words go together, and if there was any other measure by which to use when deciding between one thing or the other, it's invaluable. For me personally, it was also confirmation that what I probably repeated a thousand times had actually stuck in their heads.

We've purposefully covered what I like to call the Spiritual ABC's over the last three sections. Accountability and Boundaries were explained and encouraged for use in a positive way for promoting your success in breaking free from you past pain. I'm going to flip the concept of consequences upside down, but only about halfway around. Consequences without teeth really offer little support toward your goal of healing and freedom.

Also, the truth is, consequences are usually out of your control. Criminal actions result in consequences handed out by a judge, work violations are handled by a supervisor, and family indiscretions are addressed by your wife or other members.

I can't in good conscience water down the importance of consequences. We face them every day, from wake up late, and miss work, to fail to identify our pain, and continue to live in misery. The only upside is that we really hate receiving discipline, so we try harder to remain on the rails to avoid the punishment.

> *For the moment all discipline seems painful rather than pleasant, but later it yields the peaceful fruit of righteousness to those who have been trained by it.*
> *Hebrews 12:11*

Friend, if you're like me, we reach a point in our misery that the consequences no longer matter. The pain is so great and the need to numb it is so intense that you almost find yourself wanting to get busted in hopes it goes away. We get to a level where we've been hurting for so long that no consequence short of death could make us feel any worse about ourselves.

That's a very dangerous point to fall into. I know; I was there. The problem we face is that we've fought to survive the pain, so there's been a resilience developed over the years. Our weakness has been calloused over for so long that besides being numb, we also become very hardened. The most hurtful thing becomes the reality that we're trapped in that lifestyle, and no matter how bad we want to do better, to feel better, to be better — we can't.

After the defeat of our spirit and the surrender to living a life controlled by our past pain and current efforts to avoid it, how do we use consequences to our benefit? There are certain influencers that motivate us in everything we do. We're here and committed to this plan because we need answers, explanations and motivations to finally break free and stay free from our past pains.

There are two ways to best use the concept of consequences, since the reality of it has little bearing in our life; or even death. Consider what our actions do to others. Start with a series of concentric circles. Maybe the outside circle includes your work acquaintances. The next ring holds your friends, while the one inside of that includes extended family. Next would maybe be your kids, and the one after that is your wife. Of course, the smallest and most affected circle is you.

While you can cross out the inner most circle representing yourself because consequences don't move you to change, how about looking at all of the other people in our lives who get screwed over because we can't pull it together. I'd suggest you actually draw out this visual. It's stunning when you actually see that there's more than just you invested in your healing.

The other option for helping the concept of consequences to maintain a sense of value in your life is to understand that the entirety of your life is the consequence of other people failing you. This may be the only way for you to comprehend the bigness of just how important consequences are. I'm not trying to lay a guilt trip on you, but I don't want to give up on helping you to pierce your heart for the reality of cause and effect.

Because your life represents the consequences of someone failing or harming you, the life of pain and dysfunction has become your normal. Suffering like we do is not normal, nor is it scriptural. You do not have to accept the life you live as all you can experience. God created us for so much more. You are not at all responsible for the harm done to you, but you are responsible for how you respond to it.

Don't allow the consequences of pain, shame and guilt take God's glory away from you.

Call To Action

1. Write out in detail what you understand the consequences of failing to heal from your past pain will do to your life.

2. Write out in detail the last consequence you paid as a result of trying to deal with your past pain.

3. Create the drawing described in the content and include as many circles with names affixed as your life connects to.

29

RESTORATION

But the one who looks into the perfect law, the law of liberty, and perseveres, being no hearer who forgets but a doer who acts, he will be blessed in his doing.
James 1:25

We've come a long way together. If you've powered through each of these last 29 days without stopping—Great Going.

If you had one or a few stops along the way thanks to that old thing we call life—Great Going.

The point is, it's day 29 and whether it's taken 29 days or a year and 29 days, all that matters is that you are here. Breaking free from our past is a process. It involves so many things, but healing freedom is our goal.

It's important to understand that there are two types of healing used by God. One is the miracle. It's an instant, in the blink of an eye type of restorative healing that is only capable by God. The other healing is a process. This takes time, patience and persistent faith. It's often used by God to draw out certain flaws or strengthen certain characteristics in the sufferer and their close allies. It's not nearly as immediate as a miracle, but the end result is just as solid.

Healing is also about restoration. There are various types of restoration, and the act of restoring us is a vibrant dynamic. One definition of the word restoration is "the action of returning something to a former owner, place, or condition." Another is "the process of repairing or renovating a building, work of art, vehicle, etc., so as to restore it to its original condition."

Do either of those apply to you? In our restoration, we are being returned to our original owner: God. A crafty car thief can steal your ride, change the VIN numbers and apply for a new title, but that still doesn't make it his car. Maybe we'd taken possession of our own lives and walked away with the deed and title, but self-ownership wasn't what was intended when the creator crafted us for this life.

The other definition describes being repaired and renovated, so as to restore to its original condition. I love how this secular definition fits so perfect into God's design. Our original condition was Adam. Honestly, we've moved the needle a long way from those earliest days walking nude with lions. But, thanks be to Christ's sacrifice for our salvation, He is the second Adam, and thus a hope restored for living a Christlike life; Christian.

I talk with people all the time that feel as though they lose a layer of who they are each time they sin and ask for forgiveness. It takes them a while if ever to understand that when God forgives them, they are fully restored. As in the old hymn, *What Can Wash Away My Sin?* They aren't almost white as snow, or beige or even eggshell, we are washed white as snow.

> *What can wash away my sin? Nothing but the blood of Jesus; What can make me whole again? Nothing but the blood of Jesus.*
> *Oh! precious is the flow That makes me white as snow; No other fount I know, Nothing but the blood of Jesus.*

Let's also be very blunt at this point. There are some who assume because they are forgiven of sin, that it's a blank check to live as they wish, and sin again because they know God will forgive them again and again and again.

Being forgiven by God requires more than a plea in a time of panic. God demands confession, repentance and a contrite heart toward change. If you ask forgiveness because you feel sad over what you did or got caught doing; and not because of the hurt you caused others and pain brought to God, then you are still beyond the spiritual realm of God's loving nature.

Restoration is such a vital word in this conversation, because it's exactly the process of not only being washed white as snow of your transgressions, but returning to the original owner and creator, God. That is forgiveness and restoration.

Restoration is where we want to be, and where we want to stay. Adam was in paradise in God's presence in what we know was the Garden of Eden. He was provided everything including the intimacy of Eve. Sin for them, just like for us, separated us all from God's presence.

How drastically different do you think Adam's life was without God's constant presence and relationship? How different are our lives while in the midst of the sin we commit thanks often to carrying around our past pain? Through restoration we have been given the gift to draw near our Father once again. Yes, we've experienced pain in our lives even while we walked by His side, but that pain is for us to process.

God knows our hearts but won't force Himself into it without our invitation. That even goes for the most ardent believer. He is actively waiting to come it, but we must be open to restoration.

Behold, I stand at the door, and knock: if any man hear my voice, and open the door, I will come in to him, and will sup with him, and he with me.
Revelation 3:20

We've come so far in this process. There have been days I know you might've just closed the cover and moved on, but there was also something that said, "Don't quit." That's the voice of God, and you are hearing it because He loves you and doesn't want to lose you any longer than He already has.

Our pain, while mostly came as a result of someone else's sin, has caused us to branch off into sinful behavior while fighting to combat the pain from our past. This is our time to close the gap and restore life as God intended it to be lived.

Repent therefore, and turn back, that your sins may be blotted out, that times of refreshing may come from the presence of the Lord, and that he may send the Christ appointed for you, Jesus,
Acts 3:19-20

Call To Action

1. Write out in detail about something that you have restored. Maybe it was a car, furniture, a picture, a hobby, or a relationship. How did it make you feel?

2. Write out in detail what it is that is broken in your life, and in need of God to restore back to its glory.

3. Write out in detail sinful behaviors that you still struggle with, and your plan to commit them to God for repair and restoration.

4. Write out in detail what you envision a restored you to look like.

30

REMAINING FREE

And you will know the truth, and the truth will set you free.
John 8:32

This is always the hardest part to pen. There is so much that goes into writing these books, that instead of the end being the end, it is actually a new beginning. I learn so much during the process and am overwhelmed through prayers and memories of my own struggles. Sharing scenarios I dealt with on my path to breaking free from the pain of my past now brings more joy than darkness. For that I am grateful, and I pray that over you as well.

I don't think you ever "get over it," by pushing it to the back of your mind, or simply forgetting about it. Your past is a part of who you were, are and will be. Like an injury scar to the body, it'll fade, but the cause of the scar no longer is the emergency it once was when you needed medical attention.

So, as I wrote each section, some days took longer because the memories and emotions became too strong to keep writing through. That didn't mean I wasn't healed, it just meant I was human and no longer had to hide the way I felt about what had happened. This is the point I pray you're at or soon will reach. Healing is a process, and the length of the process is up to you. I recall as my wife and I sat in a Christian marriage counselor's office, I asked him how long the process would take. He said the average was about five years. I laughed and said, I'll beat that. The reality is, it'll take as long as the effort you are willing to put into it.

This book is so personal to me, that I truly am thankful you've allowed me to work with you in your commitment to gain freedom from your past of personal pain. It not only changed, but also saved my life. I want you to be where I am too. There is nothing like the taste of freedom.

So many loved ones, friends and acquaintances are pulling for you. The new you will also see how many other opportunities for getting back into a healthy, intentional life are waiting down the line.

This is a tough challenge, so I pray you know what you've just accomplished. It's not easy to look at ourselves without blinking or making excuses for the bad behavior we've engaged in because of what someone or something did to us in our past. I've said it earlier; but while you are not responsible for what was done to you in your past, you are responsible for how now you respond to it.

Powering through this tough look at yourself and the circumstances of your life, is taking that responsibility for it now. You've made a statement to yourself, and most importantly to God, that you will pursue and cling to Him for your freedom. No one I know has been freed and stayed free without Jesus Christ as the lead in their life. Stick to the Rock.

And, speaking of the Rock, I want to share my blessing with you. Jesus Christ has been so good to me but keeping the anointing oil in my jar isn't fulfilling His calling to anoint others with God's healing grace. I prayed over every section before I began to write, and I'll continue to pray for everyone who has read this book. There is healing to be gained, my friend.

God transcends what we understand as chronological time. He moves back and forth and side to side within our continuum. God has placed your blessing at a certain point in time, and it is waiting for you to continue pressing forward to claim it. That gift is freedom from all that haunts you. That freedom will bless you with a realistic view of your past life, and an optimistic view of your future.

I'm so fired up about what your future holds in store.

Rak Chazak Amats!!!

This ancient Hebrew war cry has emboldened God's warriors for centuries. The call to be strong, courageous and without hesitation to consider the impossibilities makes conquerors of us all.

I love the rally speeches that fire people up to victory. Be it a game of sandlot baseball or a battlefield, we fight for each other and something bigger than ourselves. This Hebrew call to victory has launched many God-inspired warriors into battle. May it now lead you.

"Be strong and courageous. Do not be afraid or terrified because of them, for the Lord your God goes with you; he will never leave you nor forsake you." Then Moses summoned Joshua and said to him in the presence of all Israel, "Be strong and courageous, for you must go with this people into the land that the Lord swore to their ancestors to give them, and you must divide it among them as their inheritance.
The Lord himself goes before you and will be with you; he will never leave you nor forsake you. Do not be afraid; do not be discouraged."
Deuteronomy 31:6-8

Can you imagine living life with this stamped on our hearts? No enemy too big, too strong, too intimidating. No calling of God too big, too bold, too demanding.

Joshua 1 tells about God's command to Joshua before he leads the nation into the promise land. There were still enemies trying to occupy what God had promised, but He assured Joshua of his success and inspired him to not be afraid, or discouraged, but rather be strong and courageous because God was with him.

"Have I not commanded you? Be strong and courageous. Do not be afraid; do not be discouraged, for the Lord your God will be with you wherever you go."
Joshua 1:9

God is with you, and your promised land is a life free from a painful past, and a future blessing of basking within the light of God's will. But first, you, just like I did, and Joshua did, must confront and slay your enemies who threaten to keep you away from God's promise.

Guess what? Nothing you've been through or are going through is unknown to God. You've lived through each and every one of your worst days in life and you are still here. It's not ever too hard, too tough, or too deep for God to rescue you from it. But, like Jesus says in Revelation 3:20:

Here I am! I stand at the door and knock. If anyone hears my voice and opens the door, I will come in and eat with that person, and they with me.
Revelation 3:20

Knock, call, or cry out to Jesus, and He is there with you. No pride. No ego. No shame. Only Freedom. It is yours, if you're just willing to march forward with *Rak Chazk Amats*. We've got to armor ourselves and stand the gap for Christ. When the devil unleashes his wicked attacks, we will be ready with the war cry:

> *Rak Chazak Amats!*
> *Rak Chazak Amats!!*
> *Rak Chazak Amats!!!*

See you in the trenches,
Scott

Call To Action

1. Write out in detail what it means to you to have finished these last 30 days.

2. Write out in detail what the next 30 days in your life will look like.

3. Write out in detail a letter to yourself telling you how proud you are for finishing this challenge.

4. Pat yourself on the back, and whisper, "Rak Chazak Amats."

DR. SCOTT SILVERII

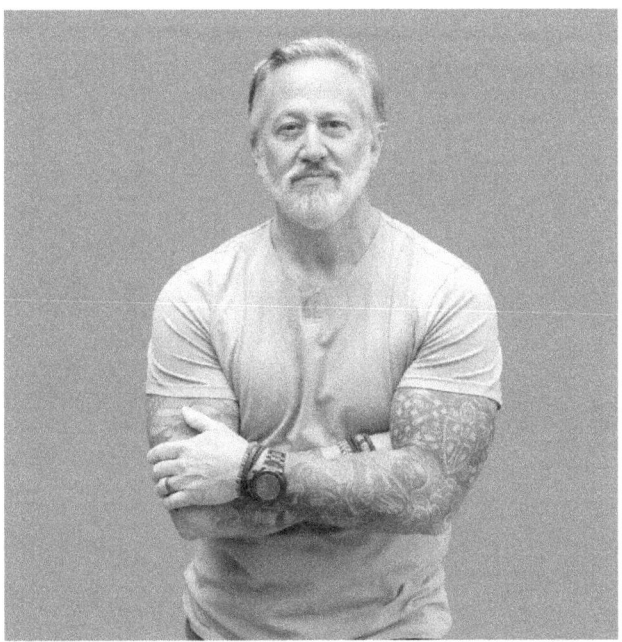

Dr. Scott Silverii is a son of the Living God. Thankful for the gift of his wife, Leah, they share seven kids, a French bulldog named Bacon and a micro-mini Goldendoodle named Biscuit.

A highly decorated, twenty-five-year law enforcement career promptly ended in retirement when God called Scott out of public service and into HIS service. The "Chief" admits that leading people to Christ is more exciting than the twelve years he spent undercover, sixteen years in SWAT, and five years as chief of police combined.

Scott has earned post-doctoral hours in a Doctor of Ministry degree in addition to a Master of Public Administration and a Ph.D. in Cultural Anthropology. Education and experience allow for a deeper understanding in ministering to the wounded, as he worked to break free from his own past pain and abuse.

In 2016, Scott was led to plant a church. Exclusive to online ministry, Five Stones Church.Online was born out of the calling to combat the negative influences reigning over social media. Scott's alpha manhood model for heroes is defined by, "Be on your guard; stand firm in the faith; be courageous; be strong. Do everything in love." (1 Corinthians 16:13-14)

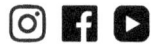

ALSO BY DR. SCOTT SILVERII

Favored Not Forgotten: Embrace the Season, Thrive in Obscurity, Activate Your Purpose

Unbreakable: From Past Pain To Future Glory

Retrain Your Brain - Using Biblical Meditation To Purify Toxic Thoughts

God Made Man - Discovering Your Purpose and Living an Intentional Life

Captive No More - Freedom From Your Past of Pain, Shame and Guilt

Broken and Blue: A Policeman's Guide To Health, Hope, and Healing

Life After Divorce: Finding Light In Life's Darkest Season

Police Organization and Culture: Navigating Law Enforcement in Today's Hostile Environment

The ABCs of Marriage: Devotional and Coloring Book

Love's Letters (A Collection of Timeless Relationship Advice from Today's Hottest Marriage Experts)

A First Responder Devotional

40 Days to a Better Firefighter Marriage

40 Days to a Better Military Marriage

40 Days to a Better Corrections Officer Marriage

40 Days to a Better 911 Dispatcher Marriage

40 Days to a Better EMT Marriage

40 Days to a Better Police Marriage

PAYING IT FORWARD

- Watch each other's back!
    - Share Captive No More with others.
    - Leave a review online wherever you bought this book.
    - Post the book and buy links on your social media so others find the help they need.
    - Message me for interviews, speaking, blog tour or questions. Personal email - scottsilverii@gmail.com
    - Be the incredible human God created you to be!

ACKNOWLEDGMENTS

I give all glory and praise to my heavenly Father. It was His son, Jesus Christ who lifted me up when I wanted to stay down, and the Holy Spirit who now pours life into my soul so that I may pour out into others.

I want to thank my loving *ezer*, Leah and our wonderfully blended family of kids and a French Bulldog, Bacon.

A special appreciation to my editor, Imogen Howson, and cover artist Darlene Albert of Wicked Smart Design.

www.ingramcontent.com/pod-product-compliance
Lightning Source LLC
Chambersburg PA
CBHW062038120526
44592CB00035B/1254

Proverbs

3:7 3:7 3:34 4:18 6:16-17 8:13 8:13 8:13 9 10:32 14:21 14:31 16:6 16:32 17:3 17:27 20:17 20:17 21:26 24:12 25:2 25:24 26:11 26:12 28:13 28:14 28:14 30:2-4 30:5-6 30:32

Ecclesiastes

10:2-3 11:5 12:14

Song of Solomon

1:3 1:4 1:15 2:5 2:11-12 2:14 3:1-2 3:11 5:8 6:8 7:2 7:11-12 8:6 8:11-12

Isaiah

1:12-15 1:16 1:18 1:19 2:10 2:11-17 2:19 2:21 5:1-8 5:21 6 6:3 11:3 11:6-9 14:23-24 19:18 26:8 26:10 27:2-3 32 32:6 33:7 35:8 35:8 35:8 35:10 38:3 40:13 43:22 45:29 48:1-2 52:1 52:7 53:8 55 55:7 57:1 57:5 57:15 57:15 58 58:2 61:1-2 63:15 63:17 64:5 64:5 65:5 65:5 65:25 66:1-2 66:2 66:2 66:5 66:5

Jeremiah

1:6 3:10 3:23-25 4:2 4:3-4 5:7 7:11 12:16 13:17 17:7 17:7-8 17:9-10 17:10 17:13 22:15-16 22:16 22:16 22:16 32:19

Lamentations

1:17 3:28

Ezekiel

3:7 3:20 9:4 11:19 13:7 16:6 16:56 16:60 16:61 16:63 18:24 20:38 20:41-42 20:42-43 33:1 33:12-13 33:13 33:20 33:31-32 36:26 44:6-7

Daniel

3:28-30 4:1-3 4:1-3 4:13 4:17 4:23 4:34 4:34-35 4:35 4:37 4:37 6:25 6:25-27 10 10:8 12:10 12:10

Hosea

4:16 6:6 6:6 7:8 10:4 13:1 13:1 14:9

Joel

3:17

Micah

6:8   6:8   6:8

Habakkuk

2:4   3:16   3:16

Zechariah

9:9   12:12-14   13:4   13:9   13:9   14:21

Malachi

1:13   3:3

Matthew

3:6   3:7-9   3:8   3:8   3:10   3:10   3:12   5:3   5:4   5:4   5:5   5:6   5:7
5:7   5:7   5:9   5:12   5:12   5:15-16   5:16   5:29-30   5:29-30   5:45-46
5:46   6:5-6   6:6   6:12   6:14   6:15   6:16   6:17   7:16   7:19-20   8:4
8:20   8:24-26   9:8   9:13   9:36   10:22   10:39   10:42   11   11:27
11:28-29   11:29   12:7   12:43-45   12:49-50   13:4-8   13:19-23   13:20
13:26   14:14   15:22   15:26-28   15:31   15:32   16:15-17   16:16-17
16:23   16:27   18   18:3   18:3-4   18:4   18:6   18:22   18:31   19:14
19:16   21:5   22:37-40   22:39-40   23:6-7   23:23   24:10-13   24:12-13
24:12-13   25   25   25   25:8   25:26   25:30   25:31   26:1   26:41
26:75   28:8   28:8   28:9   34

Mark

1:4   2:12   3:5   3:5   6:20   6:34   6:34   8:38   9:24   10:15   10:15
11:25-26   14:72

Luke

1:53   2:27   4:15   5:26   5:27-28   6:23   6:32   6:44   7   7   7:13   7:16
7:37   8:13   8:43-44   9:55   9:62   10:3   10:21-22   11:52   12:35
12:57   13:6   13:26   14:7   14:10   15   15:18   17:32   18   18:9   18:11
19:16-23   19:41-42   22:15   22:28   22:62   24:32   24:32   24:49

John

1:14   1:14   1:16   1:16   1:34   2:17   2:23-25   3:6   3:6   3:11   3:29
4:14   4:14   4:14   4:14   4:14   4:32   4:34   4:34   5:35   5:35   5:35
5:36   5:42   6   6:40   6:40   6:40   6:40   6:45   6:47   6:50-51   6:54
6:58   6:68-69   7:37-39   7:38-39   8:30-31   8:31   9:40   11   11:25
12:18   12:19   12:40   12:45   13:17   13:33   13:34   14   14   14:2
14:16-17   14:17   14:21   14:21   15:1   15:1-2   15:4   15:5   15:6   15:6-8   15:8   15:10   15:11   15:14   15:16   16:27   17:6-8   17:6-8   17:8
17:13   17:21   17:26   19:9   20   20:22   20:29   21:15

Acts

1:4   2:38   2:38-39   2:41   2:46-47   3:14   4:13   4:21   4:27   4:34-35
8:13   8:23   8:37   10:22   13:48   14:3   19:9   20:19   20:19   22:3
22:14-15   26:20   26:25

Romans

1:9   1:11   1:21   2:5   2:6   2:6   2:7   2:13   2:19-20   2:20   2:29   2:31
4:1-2   5:2-3   5:3   5:5   6:3-8   7:4-9   7:13   7:19   7:25   8   8:1   8:6
8:6   8:6-7   8:9   8:9-11   8:10   8:14   8:15-17   8:16   8:16   8:22   8:24
8:24   8:29   8:36   9:2   9:18   10:2   10:2   11:20   12:1   12:1-2   12:2
12:11   12:15   12:16   13:7   13:8   13:8   13:8-10   13:10   13:14   14:6
14:11

1 Corinthians

1:8-9   1:27-29   2:4   2:12   2:13-14   2:14   2:14   2:14   2:14   2:14-15
3   3:2   3:16   4:5   4:20   6:9-10   6:17   6:17   8:2   9:2   9:25-26   9:26
9:26   11:15   13   13:1-3   13:2   13:2   13:4   13:4-5   13:6   13:8-12
13:10-11   13:13   14:20   15:47-49

2 Corinthians

1:1   1:8-10   1:12   1:12   1:12   1:19   1:22   1:22   1:22   1:24   1:29
2:4   2:4   2:4   2:14   2:14   3:18   3:18   3:18   4:3-4   4:3-6   4:5   4:6
4:7   4:18   5:5   5:5   5:5   5:7   5:10   5:14-15   5:16-17   6:10   6:11
6:16   7:4   7:7   7:9   7:13   7:15   7:15   7:16   8:2   8:2   8:8   8:8   8:16
10:5   11:2-3   12:6   12:9   12:19   13:5

Galatians

1:14   1:14   1:16   1:16   2:20   2:20   2:20   2:20   2:20   3:1   3:13-14
3:14   3:15   4:6   4:11   4:15   4:15   4:19   5   5:14   5:14   5:14   5:16
5:18   5:21   6:1   6:4   6:7   6:7   6:9

Ephesians

1:1   1:3   1:4   1:13   1:13   1:13-14   1:14   1:14   1:16   1:17-20   1:18-19   3:7   3:7   3:17-19   3:20   4:4   4:11-12   4:13   4:16   4:22-24   5:5-6   5:21   6:1   6:5   6:5   6:24

Philippians

1:4   1:8   1:8   1:9   1:20   1:21   2:1   2:1   2:3   2:7   2:10-11   2:12   2:12   2:21   2:21   3:1   3:3   3:6   3:7   3:7-8   3:8   3:13   3:13-15   3:18-19   4:1   4:1-2   4:10

Colossians

1:9   1:9   1:9   1:22-23   1:29   1:34   2:1   2:2   2:18   2:18   2:23   3:7-8   3:10   3:10   3:12   3:12   3:12-13

1 Thessalonians

1:3   1:5   2:2   2:6   2:7-8   2:8   3:9   5:8   5:16

2 Thessalonians

1:1   1:4

1 Timothy

1:5   2:9   3   4   5   6:6

2 Timothy

1:4   1:7   1:7   1:12   1:12   1:12   2:15   3:5   3:5   4:4-8   4:6-7   4:7-8

Titus

1:1   1:16   2:14   2:14   2:14   3:3

Philemon

1:1   1:5   1:12   1:20

Hebrews

2:4   3:6   3:6   3:8   3:12   3:14   6   6:4-5   6:4-6   6:7-8   6:9-10   6:11-12   6:11-12   6:17-18   6:18   6:19   9:9   10:22   10:35   10:36   11:1

11:1 11:1 11:1 11:3 11:8 11:8-9 11:13 11:17 11:23 11:27
11:29 11:36 12:1 12:1 12:10 12:10 13:9

James

1:2-3 1:2-3 1:12 1:15 1:19 1:25 1:26 1:27 1:27 2 2:13-16
2:18 2:21-24 2:22 3:1-2 3:14-17 3:17

1 Peter

1:3 1:6 1:6-7 1:7 1:7 1:8 1:13-14 2:2-3 2:2-3 2:17 2:18
3:2 3:15 4:14 5:5 5:12

1 John

1:3 1:3 2:3 2:3 2:3 2:3 2:3 2:4-5 2:9-10 2:19 2:20 2:20
2:27 3:3 3:3 3:6 3:7-8 3:9 3:14 3:16 3:17 3:18-19 3:19-21
4:7 4:12 4:13 4:13-15 4:14 4:15 4:15 4:16 4:16 4:18 4:18
4:18 4:19 5:3 5:3 5:8 5:10

2 John

1:6 1:6

3 John

1:3 1:3-6 1:11

Jude

1:3 1:4 1:12 1:13 1:19

Revelation

1 1:17 2:7 2:10 2:10 2:13 2:17 2:17 2:17 2:17 2:23 2:23
2:26 3:1 3:7 3:10 3:12 3:15-16 3:17-18 3:19 4:8 7:3 14:4
14:10 20:12 21:6 21:6 21:6-7 21:27 22:1 22:12 22:17 40:22

Jonathan Edwards

Jonathan Edwards